Rosemary Oil

Other titles in Thorsons Aromatherapy Series:

Aromatherapy and the Mind
Aromatherapy for Lovers
Aromatherapy for Women
Aromatherapy Massage
Aromatherapy Workbook
Creative Aromatherapy
The Fragrant Year
Holistic Aromatherapy
Practical Aromatherapy

By the same author:

Aromatherapy and the Mind
The Illustrated Encyclopaedia of Essential Oils
(Element Books)
Home Aromatherapy (Kyle Cathie)
Lavender Oil
Rose Oil
Tea Tree Oil

Rosemary Oil

**THE NEW GUIDE TO NATURE'S
MOST REVITALIZING REMEDY**

Julia Lawless

To Judy

Thorsons
An Imprint of HarperCollins*Publishers*
77–85 Fulham Palace Road,
Hammersmith, London W6 8JB

1160 Battery Street,
San Francisco, California 94111-1213

Published by Thorsons 1996
1 3 5 7 9 10 8 6 4 2

A catalogue record for this book
is available from the British Library

ISBN 0 7225 3349 7

Printed in Great Britain by
Caledonian International Book Manufacturing Ltd, Glasgow

Contents

dizziness; fever; flu; gout; hair care; hangover;
headaches; immune system (to strengthen); insect
repellent; jetlag; laryngitis; liver problems/congestion;
low blood-pressure (hypotension); lumbago; migraine;
mouth and gum infections; muscular aches and pains;
neuralgia; oedema (fluid retention); palpitations
(tachycardia); perfume; perspiration (excessive);
pets/animal care; rheumatism; sciatica; sinusitis;
skin care; sore throat; sprains; stress; varicose veins;
whooping cough

Acknowledgements

> This common Rosemary is so well knowne through all
> our land, being in every woman's garden, that it were
> sufficient but to name it as an ornament among other
> sweete herbes and flowers in our Garden
>
> John Parkinson, Paradisus in Sole/Paradisis Terrestris
>
> (1629)

When I began writing this book I had only one rosemary bush (*Rosmarinus officinalis var. officinalis*) growing in the kitchen garden. Over the last few months, however, my collection of herbs has expanded to include several species of rosemary, including the beautiful deep-blue 'Severn Sea' variety. Apart from its value for its essential oil, rosemary is one of the most versatile and pleasing aromatic plants to grow. As an evergreen it keeps its form all year round, while the fresh 'needles' are always available for cooking. Even when dried, the leaves retain the most delightful and enduring scent. Like lavender and rose, it is one of the quintessential garden shrubs.

This book is dedicated to Judith Allan, with whom I have shared an ever-increasing enthusiasm for gardening

— especially with regard to herbs and fragrant plants. Over the past few years she has also given me encouragement as a writer, and we have worked on several projects together. I am grateful to the editor of *Current Research on Medicinal and Aromatic Plants* for permission to include 'The Chemistry of Rosemary Oil: A Review' — see Appendix B. I would also like to thank Cara Denman, Wanda Whiteley and those at Thorsons, as well as my husband Alec and daughter Natasha, for their ongoing support.

Rosemary Oil: An Introduction

Rosemarie, the chiefest beauties of Gardens and not to
be wanted in the Kitchen.

B. Googe, *Four Books of Husbandry* (1577)

Rosemary has been called the 'Prince' of aromatic
herbs — and it is not difficult to understand why! This
handsome evergreen shrub with narrow, dark green
leaves and small blue or mauve flowers has been cultivated since ancient times and is still a familiar sight in
many gardens today. The flowers and 'needles' are
endowed with the most delightful, refreshing scent,
and rosemary has always been valued as one of the most
important culinary herbs, having a strong, distinctive
flavour. It has also been highly esteemed for its medicinal and cosmetic properties for thousands of years, and
once played a central role in many traditional rites and
ceremonies.

Rosemary belongs to the large botanical family *Labi-
atae* (*Lamiaceae*) along with lavender and many of the
other common aromatic herbs, including marjoram,
sage, thyme and mint. The native habitat of the wild
rosemary (*Rosmarinus officinalis*) is Asia Minor and

southern Europe; like lavender, it thrives in the Mediterranean region. It can still be found growing in profusion along the Mediterranean coastline, on the Balkan Peninsula, throughout Spain and Portugal and, to a lesser extent, in Turkey, Egypt and the Lebanon. It is one of the few shrubs that can survive the rigorous climate of the Sahara desert, although it is more at home growing in proximity to water. Indeed, its name is derived from the Latin *ros* (dew) and *marinus* (sea), meaning 'Dew of the Sea'.

Rosemary has probably been cultivated in Great Britain for over 600 years, having been introduced by the Romans. Some sources say that it then went out of cultivation until the fourteenth century, when it was re-introduced by Queen Philippa, wife of King Edward III. Today it can be found growing in gardens through-out the world, even as far north as Canada, Scandinavia and Russia. In more northerly climes, however, it rarely grows taller than 1.2 m (4 ft) high, whereas in its natural habitat *Rosmarinus officinalis* can reach 1.8 m (6 ft) or more in height. It is also slightly frost-tender and needs the protection of a cold frame or the shelter of a south- or west-facing wall to survive a cold winter. Neither will rosemary tolerate water-logged condi-tions, and is best grown in well-drained limey soil or in a pot containing lots of broken crockery to ensure good drainage.

Rosemary is a favourite with gardeners and is often grown purely as a decorative plant both for its scent and for its fine stature. Gertrude Jekyll writes in her book *House and Garden* '... ever-blessed rosemary all over the garden, so that at every few steps the passer-by can run his hand over the blue-flowered branchlets and smell the warm resinous incense in his palm.'

Sir Thomas More let it run all over his garden walls because, he wrote, 'My bees love it.' Other men have apparently been more cautious about letting it grow too freely! There is an old folk belief that says 'where rosemary flourishes, the woman rules':

> There is a vulgar belief in Gloucestershire and other coun-
> ties, that Rosemary will not grow well unless where the
> mistress is 'master'; and so touchy are some of the lords of
> creation upon this point, that we have more than once had
> reason to suspect them of injuring a growing rosemary in
> order to destroy this evidence of their want of authority.[1]

There are now many different cultivars or species available to the gardener, each with differing flower and leaf colours. The flowers can be bright blue, purplish-blue, pink, white, pale mauve or a soft, powdery blue. The needle-like leaves can vary from a dull, dark green to a variegated silver or golden form. However, the green-leaved common rosemary (*R. officinalis var. officinalis*) is the only type used medicinally and is the variety usually employed for the production of essential oil. It is also generally the type used for cooking.

Other well-known cultivars, some of which are occasionally used for essential oil production, include:

Rosmarinus officinalis var. *albus*: the white-flowered variety, quite rare

R. officinalis var. *argenteus*: a rare silver-leaved variegated form

R. officinalis var. *aureus*: a half-hardy, golden-leaved variegated form

R. officinalis 'Benenden Blue' (sometimes known as 'Blue Lagoon': green-leaved with bright blue flowers

R. officinalis var. *fastigiatus* 'Miss Jessup's Upright': an erect, compact shrub often grown as a hedge

R. officinalis var. *roseus*: a form with rosy-pink flowers

R. officinalis var. *lavandulaceus (procumbens)*: a tender, low-growing species sometimes used for the production of an essential oil

R. officinalis 'Severn Sea': a decorative species with brilliant blue flowers

R. officinalis var. *angustifolia (tenuifolius)*: a pine-scented species occasionally used for the production of an essential oil.

PART I

A Medical and
Historical Background

CHAPTER ONE

The Herb of Remembrance

There's rosemary, that's for remembrance;
pray you love, remember ...

Hamlet, IV.v

In Ophelia's well-known parting words to Hamlet, rosemary is associated with enduring love and faithfulness, even beyond the grave. In the so-called 'language of flowers' which was popular in Europe during the Middle Ages, rosemary stood for 'remembrance' and, in Shakespeare's time, the symbolic significance of many flowers and herbs was still common knowledge. Yet rosemary has been linked with the rituals of both marriage and death since antiquity, through the common theme of 'remembrance' or 'undying devotion'.

Grow it for two ends, it matters not at all
Be't for my bridall or my buriall ...

Robert Herrick, *Book of Rosemary*

Rosemary's associations with funeral rites go back to the time of the ancient Egyptians: traces of the dried herb have been found in First Dynasty tombs (circa

2000 BC). The archaeologist Prospero Alpini found sprigs of rosemary within the wrappings of a mummy in Cairo, which suggests it was used as part of the embalming process. This also gives an indication of rosemary's preservative properties and why it became such an important culinary herb, especially in those times when food needed to be stored without the luxury of refrigeration.

> For you there's rosemary and rue; these keep
> Seeming and savour all winter long:
> Grace and remembrance be to you both
>
> *The Winter's Tale*, Act IV.iii

As an evergreen plant which retained its fragrance for longer than most other herbs once picked and dried, and since it could be used to preserve other foods, rosemary became a fitting emblem for loyalty and steadfastness. It was often used as a Christmas decoration or given as a New Year's gift, together with an orange stuck with cloves, as a sign of regeneration. Such qualities also helped to give rosemary the reputation for preserving youth and promoting longevity: 'Make thee a box of the wood and smell it and it shall preserve thy youth...'[1]

The ancient Romans employed the herb in their bath houses for maintaining a glowing complexion and toning the muscles, while for the Greeks the scent of rosemary was thought to stimulate the intellect and keep the mind alert. Greek students would consequently wear a wreath of rosemary in their hair when taking examinations, to improve their memory. The ancient Greeks also used rosemary in the form of incense at religious ceremonies, especially during funerals, when prepared incense was not available. Later it became traditional to place a wreath of rosemary on the grave of a loved one, to show that the dead would not be forgotten. Within the Christian tradition, these wreathes subsequently became a sign of Christ's faithful promise of resurrection, and until quite recently it was customary in Wales to strew sprigs of rosemary onto the coffin of a deceased loved one before it was covered with earth. Sir Thomas More wrote: 'It is the herb sacred to remembrance, and, therefore to friendship; whence a sprig of it hath a dumb language that maketh it the chosen emblem of our funeral wakes and in our burial grounds.'[2]

As a symbol of remembrance, rosemary was just as popular at weddings as at funerals. In Europe during the Middle Ages, the herb was used as a marriage decoration, and was traditionally included in the bride's bouquet or worn in her crown as a sign of fidelity. Anne of Cleves wore rosemary in her coronet at her marriage to Henry VIII, and all her wedding chests were said to have been made from rosemary wood. Another custom of that time demanded that during the ceremony each member of the bridal party should hold a sprig of rosemary in her right hand as testimony that the bride was still a virgin. Even as late as the nineteenth century it was common for women to include a few sprigs of rosemary in their wedding posy.

> The bride was led to church between two sweet boys
> with bridelaces and Rosemary tied to their silken sleeves.[3]

After the marriage, the bed linen was scented with
dried rosemary, and the bride who gave her husband a
sprig to hold on their wedding night would ensure that
he remained faithful. Another way of preventing the
groom from straying from the marriage bed was to
place three rosemary leaves in the Bible at the passage
from 'The Song of Solomon' that reads 'Let him always
kiss her with the kisses of his mouth' and then put the
Bible under his pillow. According to another old folk
saying, which would seem more useful *before* marriage
than afterwards, if a man doesn't like the smell of rosemary he will be no good in bed!

> It holds a special position among herbs from the symbol-
> ism attached to it. Not only was it used at weddings but
> also at funerals, for decking churches and banqueting
> halls at festivals, as incense in religious ceremonies, and
> in magical spells.[4]

Rosemary can also be regarded as one of the 'sacred'
herbs, which over the centuries have gathered many
legends and folk beliefs around them. The early Greeks
and Romans considered rosemary a magical plant, and
the Roman poet Horace composed odes to its super-
natural properties. In Europe during the pre-Christian

era, rosemary was carried as a protection aga.nst evil and was used in ceremonies involving purification or an exorcism of some kind. It is still a favourite herb among gypsies, who hang a bunch of rosemary by the door as a protective charm where a child is sleeping. It also acts as a charm against nightmares! As one fourteenth-century manuscript says:

> The leves layde under the head whannea man slepes, it doth away evell spirites and suffereth not to dreame fowle dremes ne to be afeade. But he must be out of deedly synne for it is an holy tree. Lavender and Rosemary is as woman to man and Whote Roose to Reede. It is an holy tree and with ffolke that been just and Rightfull gladlye it groweth and thryveth.[5]

The Spaniards call it 'Romero' – the 'Pilgrim's Flower' – and in Spain and Italy it has long been considered a safeguard against witches and evil influences, especially on long journeys. Its connection with the sea, as demonstrated by its old folk names 'Compass Plant', 'Polar Plant' and 'Compass-weed', also hint at its protective and preservative attributes. The diagram on the background of a compass showing all directions in relation to North (originally magnetic north but, later, polar north) is still called the 'mariner's rose'. The 'needle', pointing north, again indicates 'constancy' or 'loyalty'. The familiar scent of the herb growing along the Mediterranean coastline must have once welcomed sailors returning home, for the rosemary flowers were

'credibly reported to give their scent above thirty
leagues off at sea, upon the coast of Spain'.[6]

Primitive beliefs regarding the herb's protective
qualities are no doubt based largely on its excellent
antiseptic and prophylactic powers, which is why it was
also used as a preventative in times of plague during the
Middle Ages and was later burned in French hospitals
to inhibit the spread of disease. According to French
folklore, the scent of burning rosemary also renewed
one's energy and helped to stimulate the mind. Indeed,
it is a well-known fact that certain scents can enliven
the mental faculties or act as a trigger to evoke long-
forgotten memories. In the popular folk song 'Scarbor-
ough Fair', four of the most aromatic herbs, including
rosemary, are mentioned again and again in the refrain
in recollection of a past lover:

> Where are you going? To Scarborough Fair.
> Parsley, sage, rosemary and thyme,
> Remember me to a bonny lass there,
> For once she was a true lover of mine.[7]

There are also several Christian legends associated
specifically with this herb. According to one story, the
rosemary bush will grow no higher than 2 m (6 ft) tall,
so as not to exceed the height of Christ, and will only
grow in breadth after 33 years (Christ's age at the time
of his crucifixion). In another legend, the flowers of the
rosemary were originally said to be white, but were
changed to blue when the Virgin Mary threw her cloak

over the silvery bush while resting during her journey
into Egypt.

> Tansy, thyme, sweet cicely,
> Saffron, balm, and rosemary,
> That since the virgin threw her cloak,
> Across it — so say cottage folk —
> Has changed its flowers from white to blue...[8]

It is interesting to note that the mass of legends and
folklore which has gathered around rosemary over the
centuries tends to reflect the same basic elements
which are inherent in the therapeutic action of the herb
itself — as a protection against disease; as a preservative;
and as a cephalic and nerve tonic for sharpening the
mind and intellect.

CHAPTER TWO

A Traditional
'Cure All' Folk Remedy

> Speaking of the powers of rosemary, it overtoppeth all
> the flowers in the garden, boasting man's rule. It helpeth
> the brain, strengtheneth the memorie, and is very medic-
> inable for the head. Another property of the rosemary is,
> it affects the heart. Let this rosemarinus, this flower of
> men, ensigne of your wisdom, love and loyaltie, be car-
> ried not only in your hands, but in your hearts and
> heads.[1]

Rosemary is one of the native 'cure all' remedies which
can be found among the traditional folk customs of
many countries, especially those of the Mediterranean
region. It has an ancient medical history, although the
earliest record of its use specifically for therapeutic
purposes can be traced to Greek and Roman times. The
ancient Greeks burned sprigs of rosemary as an incense
on their shrines – so it became known as the 'Incense
Bush'. The great classical writers Dioscorides and
Theophrastus recommended it specifically for stomach
and liver problems. Galen too prescribed it for liver
disorders, particularly jaundice, while Hippocrates, the

'Father of Medicine', said that the herb (*R. officinalis var. officinalis*) was best cooked with vegetables to overcome liver and spleen complaints.

The Romans used infusions of rosemary for weakness of the heart, poor circulation, anaemia and nervous exhaustion. It was also employed to clean wounds and recommended for coughs and chest complaints. It was the Romans who most probably introduced rosemary to Britain, as they did in other parts of their Empire, although this was not recorded at the time. It is, however, mentioned in the Anglo-Saxon *Leech Book of Bald* (circa AD 1000) as a protection against evil spirits and as a remedy for toothache. In the thirteenth-century Myddfai manuscripts it is recommended as a charm against nightmares and 'all mental anxiety' when placed under the pillow. This tends to suggest that the herb was already in use before the fourteenth century, when the Countess of Hainault sent rosemary plants to England for her daughter Philippa, Queen of Edward III (1327–77), together with a manuscript extolling its virtues: 'Rosemary ... it mighteth the boones and causeth goode and gladeth and lighteth alle men that use it.'[2]

Throughout Europe during this period, rosemary twigs were used extensively as a fumigant in sick rooms, hospitals and as a preventative against the plague. An old French name for the herb was *Incensier*, because it was sometimes burned as incense in church. In a thirteenth-century French treatise, Arnauld de Villeneuve also describes how the essential oil could be

distilled and used as a remedy. Indeed, over the next
few centuries rosemary was one of the most valuable
medicines at the disposal of the apothecary, and was
prepared in a variety of ways. The leaves and flowers
were used fresh or dried, often mixed with wine (in the
form of a tincture) or prepared as an infusion by boiling
them in water. Aromatic oils, ointments and liniments
were commonly applied for external treatment. Rosemary was also the vital ingredient in the famous
'Queen of Hungary Water', a lotion which is said to
have completely rejuvenated and revitalized the para-
lysed limbs of that ageing sovereign. A formula dated
1235, which is thought to be in the handwriting of Elizabeth, Queen of Hungary, is still preserved in Vienna.

> It was prepared by putting one and a half pounds of fresh
> rosemary tops, in full flower [some versions include myr-
> tle and lavender] into one gallon of spirits of wine ... this
> was allowed to stand for four days and then distilled.
> Hungary water was also considered very efficacious
> against gout in the hands and feet, being rubbed into
> them vigorously.'

As a rejuvenating elixir for cosmetic purposes, rosemary was also renowned as a fine tonic for the hair and
scalp. It was used to eliminate dandruff, stimulate hair
growth, prevent baldness and generally enhance the
colour of dark hair. The doctors of Myddfai, in addition, counselled the use of rosemary for retaining a
youthful complexion:

A fine thing it is to boil in water the leaves and flowers
and to use the mixture as a face wash. Do not wipe the
face afterwards, but let it dry naturally. The truth is that
by regularly washing their faces in this way the wise will
keep their youth until the day they die.[4]

From the fifteenth to the seventeenth century, the
numerous medicinal and cosmetic applications of rosemary were duly recorded at length in the new European
herbals. Banckes' *Herbal* of 1525 gave an authoritative
list of complaints which might be treated with the herb:
'Take the flowers thereof and boyle them in fare water
and drinke that water, for it is much worthe against all
manner of evils in the body ...'[5]

Half a century later, Nicholas Culpeper (1616–54)
recommended a decoction of the herb in wine for all
'cold diseases of the head and brain', such as giddiness,
lethargy and weak memory; an infusion of the herb in
oil for rheumatism and for refining the complexion;
and that the dried leaves should be smoked in the form
of tobacco for consumption or chronic coughs.
Regarding the essential oil, he mentions the following
warning:

The chymical oil drawn from the leaves and flowers ... is
a sovereign help for all the diseases aforesaid, to touch the
temples and nostrils with two or three drops for all the
diseases of the head and brain spoken of before; as also to
take one drop, two or three, as the case requires for the
inward diseases; yet it must be done with discretion, for

it is very quick and piercing, and therefore but a little
must be taken at a time.[6]

Because of its sharp, penetrating odour, the Elizabethans used rosemary oil in place of smelling salts to
revive a faint spirit. The sixteenth and early seventeenth century also saw a revival in the use of flower
waters, which the Elizabethans used to scent their
clothes and floors, sprinkling fragrant liquids from
their 'casting bottles'. Rosemary was also a central fea-
ture in the formal Elizabethan herb gardens, where it
was often used as hedging or clipped into the shape of a
bench, a bird, a cart or some other object. In England,
as in other European countries, most large houses had
their own 'still room' where herbs could be dried and
where aromatic oils and fragrant waters could be prepared. Apart from her obsession with roses, France's
Empress Josephine is said to have loved the scent of
rosemary. She requested Napoleon to wash in rosemary water before he entered her bedchamber, and
he used it to sweeten his breath. It is recorded that
Napoleon used up 162 bottles of rosemary water in the
first three months of their marriage!

The Colonial Americans were also aware of the cosmetic benefits of rosemary, which they introduced to
the 'New World'. They used a rosemary rinse not only
to improve the shine and colour of their hair, but also
to make it curl. During the eighteenth century in the
United States, as in Europe, rosemary was also valued
as a medicine and commonly prescribed as a stimulant,

emmenagogue and anti-spasmodic, while its oil was principally employed in ointments, liniments and embrocations.

By the beginning of the nineteenth century, however, both in the US and Europe, herbal medicine was already in decline as newly discovered chemical drugs took their place. Ancient folk remedies such as rosemary lost credibility in the eyes of the professionals and public alike, while the scientific approach, with its emphasis on specialization, steadily gained ground. It was only in the first few decades of the twentieth century that the potential of plant medicines began to be re-assessed seriously in the light of new scientific evidence using modern research techniques.

CHAPTER THREE

Rosemary Oil: Chemical Analysis and Clinical Research

Forgotten and ignored for many years, aromatic essences are coming back into their own, for many researchers and for a wide section of public opinion, as the stars of medicine. Faced with a mounting toll of complications known to have been caused by aggressively synthesized chemical medications, many patients are now unwilling to be treated except by natural therapies, foremost among which plants and essences have their rightful place.[1]

The resurgence of interest in aromatherapy, medical herbalism and other natural therapies over the last few decades bears witness to the opening words of Dr Valnet's pioneering book *The Practice of Aromatherapy*, first published in France in 1964. In it, he advocates the re-evaluation of plant medicines using modern research techniques and cites many clinical tests which confirm 'the validity of traditional ideas based on practical experience'.[2]

In the past, when the chemical composition of essential oils was still a mystery, aromatic oils were used successfully to combat all types of infectious disease. Such knowledge was based on the vast accumulation of empirical evidence gathered over centuries of experimentation. In Europe during the Great Plague of 1665, for example, rosemary was burned in public places to help contain the epidemic, and was carried in special pouches or compartments inside walking sticks as protection while passing through infected areas.

Recent research has shown that rosemary is in fact one of the most potent antiseptic and prophylactic agents available. As early as the 1920s, René Gattefossé, the French chemist who first coined the term 'aromatherapie', had noted the powerful bactericidal properties of rosemary in his own clinical research based on a detailed chemical analysis of the oil:

> The essences of rosemary, sage, pine and fir contain borneol and its esters. This is what gives them their strong antiseptic qualities and accounts for their medicinal applications. Essence of rosemary is considered a beneficial stomachic against atopic dyspepsia. The leaf infusion is stimulating and has yielded excellent results for some feverish conditions causing temporary but worrying prostration.

He continues:

> Cazin obtained marvellous results for pernicious bouts of malaria. Brissemoret, in his 'Essais sur les preparations galeniques', lists it as a stimulant and tonic because of the presence of borneol, along with cam-

phor, cineol, pinene and camphene. It is a vermifuge
and an emmenagogue.[3]

Gattefossé had not been the first to draw conclusions
about the therapeutic potential of an essential oil
by examining its chemical composition. A wealth of
research had already been carried out during the previ-
ous 50 years by Calvello (1902), Marx (1903), Kobert
(1906) and Clavel (1918), to name but a few.[4] However, as a chemist with a specialist interest in aromatics
Gattefossé did make a substantial contribution to this
field, which later proved an inspiration to Dr Valnet.

Through his work as a doctor and surgeon during
the Second World War, Valnet had become especially
interested in the antiseptic properties of essential oils
and their ability to inhibit the spread of infection. He
introduced the use of natural aromatics into his clinical
practice with very successful results. In 1958 Dr Valnet
wrote: '...we learned that vapours derived from aromatic plants possess antiseptic properties which inhibit
the development of certain staphylococci and coliform
bacilli. These plants include (in descending order of
potency) thyme, rosemary, eucalyptus, peppermint,
orange blossom... etc.'[5]

To study the suppression of germs by aromatic oils
with greater precision, Valnet and his colleagues formulated a laboratory technique called the 'aromatogram'.
This method, which involved testing specific oils on
cultured bacteria *in vitro*, was used not only to ascertain
the minimum effective dosage of various oils but also

to find which one was best suited to treating a particular infection. One of the intriguing aspects of this programme was that patients responded to different oils even if suffering from the same infection! This is because, unlike antibiotics (which kill germs and healthy bacteria alike), essential oils support the body's own defence system by creating a healthy environment in which the pathogens are unable to survive – *according to the needs of each individual case*.

In 1978, Valnet and his colleagues employed the 'aromatogram' to carry out 268 test cases, using a variety of oils including rosemary. Several bacteria and fungi were tested, including *Staphylococcus aureus*, *E. coli*, *Proteus mirabilis*, *Strep. faecalis* and *Candida albicans*. Although rosemary proved to be 1.48 times more effective than antibiotics *in vitro* against the above organisms, it was not as successful as some oils, such as origanum, cinnamon, thyme or savory at combating both bacterial and fungicidal germs. Subsequent research carried out during the 1970s, eighties and early nineties has in fact confirmed that, although rosemary is effective against a wide range of bacteria, its fungicidal action is more variable:

- 1974: Opdyke – Rosemary was shown to have good antimicrobial properties in a series of tests against bacteria and fungi.[6]
- 1976: Bardeau – Several vaporized oils were tested for their capacity to destroy a range of bacteria including *Proteus*, *Staph. aureus* and *Strep. pyogenes*.

Rosemary was found to be one of the most effective essences (together with lavender, thyme, pine, marjoram and clove), and thus was found suitable for the treatment of infections such as the common cold and bronchitis.[7]

- 1987: Deans and Richie – rosemary was tested against 25 types of bacteria, and found effective against 21 varieties.[8]

- 1984: Benjilali *et al.* – rosemary and eucalyptus were demonstrated to be less effective than thyme and three artemisia oils at inhibiting 39 fungi.[9]

- 1993: Biondii *et al.* – 22 oils, including rosemary, were tested against seven bacteria. Rosemary was not among the top oils but it was noted that 'other studies gave conflicting results, and this was due to the compositional differences of the oils dependent on their source.'[10]

- 1994: Pandit and Shelef – Eighteen spices were screened for anti-listerial properties. Only rosemary and cloves were found to be listericidal.[11]

- 1995: Stellon – at the first demonstration of the aromatogram in the UK at the Royal Society of Medicine, Dr Stellon was so impressed with the results that he has begun a clinical trial comparing the effectiveness of various essential oils with antibiotics.[12] This shows a move towards re-integrating 'natural' medicines back into 'orthodox' medical practice.

'We are not talking about a complete substitute for

antibiotics', says Mr Smith (a London pathologist) ...
'on the other hand, doctors regularly prescribe an
antibiotic for something as minor as a fungal infection
of the toenail. But it makes far more sense to treat that
locally with an oil which can actually penetrate the nail,
rather than handing out a powerful drug that has known
effects on the liver and will probably knock out some of
the bacteria in your gut as well.'[13]

If the delicate balance of bacteria in the gut is
destroyed by the long-term use of antibiotics, contra-
ceptives, anti-inflammatory drugs or antacids, this can
lead to a wide range of common conditions such as irri-
table bowel syndrome, catarrh, sinusitis, cystitis or
thrush. The relationship between essential oils and the
gut is an important one, because by rebalancing the
intestinal flora using appropriate oils it becomes possible to clear up all sorts of chronic conditions. Essential oils have been prescribed in France by qualified
medical doctors for years on this basis.

Rosemary is one of the most useful oils in this context, due to its good antiseptic properties and its
affinity with the digestive tract. Valnet observed that
the intestines, 'the seat of so many troubles', were
stimulated especially by the oils of 'rosemary, cinnamon and cloves'. He also found that rosemary aided
the production and evacuation of bile and acted as a
detoxifying agent for the whole alimentary canal. In
addition: 'Rosemary oil was markedly spasmogenic
but had some spasmolytic effect also on guinea-
pig ileum *in vitro*... There was a relaxant effect on

the tracheal smooth muscle of rabbit and guinea-pig
in vitro.'[14]

The powerful antiseptic, anti-spasmodic, detoxifying
and digestive properties of *R. officinalis var. officinalis*
account for its traditional use as a culinary herb and as a
preservative. Simply using rosemary in cooking is one
way of utilizing its therapeutic properties, especially
with respect to digestive problems such as constipation
or dyspepsia. In medical herbalism, an infusion (tea) or
tincture (liquid extract in alcohol) of rosemary is still
prescribed principally for its carminative, tonic, astringent, anti-spasmodic, antimicrobial and diuretic prin-
cipals. In the *British Herbal Pharmacopoeia* it is indicated
specifically for: 'flatulent dyspepsia associated with psychogenic tension ... and depressive states with general
debility and indications of cardio-vascular weakness'.[15]

Rosemary has a long history of use as a remedy for
nervous exhaustion and general debility, having a tonic
effect on the heart and vital organs. In 1987, the stimulating properties of rosemary were demonstrated con-
clusively in a leading study conducted by Kovar *et al*.
They set out to investigate the efficiency of rosemary
oil and its main constituent (1,8-cineole), by inducing
mice to inhale its vapours. The locomotive activity of
the brain in the test animals increased significantly
when they inhaled the oil. In another experiment, a
rosmaricine derivative (0,0,N-trimethylrosmaricine)
was shown to exhibit significant smooth-muscle stimulant effects *in vitro*, as well as moderate analgesic (pain-
killing) activity. Recent research at the University of

Cincinnati and by Sugano in Japan using contingent negative variation (CNV – a device which measures electrical brainwave patterns) have shown that rosemary really can stimulate the brain and memory.[16]

In pharmaceutical work, rosemary oil is contained in a number of brands of propriety medicines for circulatory disorders and heart weakness (especially in old age), and as a tonic for the liver and gall bladder. The oil is also added to liniments to be applied topically as an analgesic and rubefacient for muscular and rheumatic pain. The cosmetics industry use the oil extensively in toothcare products, hair lotions, shampoos, soaps, bath products and skin tonics. In perfumery it is employed in the preparation of eau-de-Cologne and as an ingredient in herbaceous or chypre perfumes, such as 'Tsar'.

CHAPTER FOUR

Cultivation, Production and Quality Control

Rosemary is steam-distilled from the flowers, leaves and twigs of *Rosmarinus officinalis var. officinalis*. This method of production was first recorded in the European herbals of the Middle Ages, when the herb was held in high regard for its bactericidal properties. According to historians, rosemary oil was distilled as early as 1330 by Raymond Lully, and along with lavender was one of the first 'chymical' oils to be produced in Great Britain.[1]

Although rosemary has been grown as a herb in physic gardens for centuries and has been cultivated on a larger scale in areas such as southern France, the vast majority of essential oil is still produced from wild-growing plants. Rosemary oil is in fact one of the largest-volume herbaceous oils on the international market, with Spain, Tunisia and Morocco being the principal producers. Among the minor producers are Italy, Egypt, Portugal, Algeria, Corsica, France, and the former Yugoslavia.

The total world production of rosemary oil is in excess of 500 tonnes per year. At one time around a third of this annual production was officially exported from Spain. However, although Spain is ᛌ the largest producer it also handles a large proportion of the Moroccan oil, and some of the Tunisian exports. In Spain these imported oils are frequently blended with Spanish oil, adulterated with camphor or cineole, or simply re-labelled before being exported as 'Spanish' rosemary oil. The export figures for the true Spanish rosemary oil are therefore much smaller than is generally thought to be the case.

Today, Tunisian rosemary oil is internationally regarded as of the highest quality available on a large commercial scale, being less camphoraceous and having a more refined fragrance than the Spanish oil – as well as being less subject to adulteration! The Tunisian oil has also enjoyed a rapid increase in popularity since the early 1980s due to the perfumery industry's need for a natural anti-oxidant. Before this time a variety of chemical alternatives were used, but the flavourists and fine fragrance industries demanded a natural alternative. Specific research carried out on both *Rosmarinus* and *Salvia officinalis* resulted, in 1982, in the Department of Food and Nutrition at Osaka City University in Japan isolating one constituent – a *phenolic diterpene* – which has excellent anti-oxidant properties. The demand for this substance, which was called 'Rosemanol', soared over the next 10 years and further contributed to the decline in popularity of Spanish rosemary oil.

The Spanish and Tunisian oils vary considerably in their make-up, as is common for many essential oil-producing plants grown in different localities and climates. Indeed, great variations in the chemical composition of different oils of rosemary can be observed, due mainly to the large number of subspecies of *Rosmarinus* in use, and to the intraspecific hybridization of plants that occur in the wild and are known as 'chemotypes'. The chemical composition of an average rosemary oil is quite simple, containing about 200 main constituents. However, it is the minor constituents or trace elements which can play a major role in the overall olfactive qualities of an oil, as well as its therapeutic or medicinal potential. The following table shows a comparison of the main constituents of Tunisian and Spanish oils:

	Tunisian	Spanish
Camphor	9.9	21.8
1,8-cineole	37.6	29.6
Limonene	4.9	4.6
Borneol	4.4	3.5
Alpha pinene	11.8	20.1
Beta pinene	7.7	7.4
Camphene	4.5	4.0

(*See Appendix B* for a more detailed list of constituents.)

Indeed, there are three principal chemotypes of *R. officinalis* that can be found growing in Europe, namely the 'cineole' (Italy/Morocco), 'borneol' (Tunisia/Spain) and 'verbenone' (Algeria/Corsica) varieties.[2] Time of harvesting, condition of the plant and the type of apparatus used also play their part in the overall quality of an oil.

Ideally rosemary should be harvested when in bud, not in full flower, or the essential oil content is diminished. The plants should also be harvested on a sunny day in the morning, and subjected to distillation as soon as possible. In a typical field distillation unit, the still is fitted with a double bottom and the rosemary placed on a raised grill rather than being in direct contact with the water. This method generally yields about 0.5–1.0 per cent of oil, using fresh plant material. With a modern commercial still, on the other hand, the raw material is subjected to steam that is produced either directly or indirectly at double or triple atmospheric pressure, and distilled for about 2 to 4 hours. The oil yield in this case is about 1.0–1.5 per cent with freshly harvested plants, 1.5–2.5 per cent with dried leaves.

The essential oil obtained from fresh rosemary leaves has a camphoraceous odour with a penetrating, sharp top note. The oil obtained from the dried leaves has a fresh, herbaceous top note with a more woody/balsamic base. Other solvent extracts of the rosemary plant include an oleoresin, a concentrate, and an absolute. These are all extensively refined perfumery materials which are only produced in small quantities. A more important product is terpene-less rosemary oil, which has a more delicate scent than the standard oil and which is used in specialized pharmaceutical products and high-class perfumery.

CHAPTER FIVE

A Summary of the Properties and Applications of Rosemary Oil

In keeping with its folk reputation as a 'cure all', rosemary oil has a wide range of applications. By looking at its principal areas of action more closely, however, it is possible to divide the uses of rosemary into three main categories:

1 First and foremost it is a **tonic – a fortifying and stimulating remedy** especially with relation to the nervous and vascular (circulatory) systems.

2 Secondly it is a powerful **prophylactic agent** – that is, it has good bactericidal properties and prevents the spread of disease. It is excellent for the treatment of infectious illnesses, especially those affecting or connected with the respiratory system.

3 Thirdly, rosemary is valuable for **pain relief, bringing warmth and increased mobility** to the body, especially with regard to the muscles and joints. This is mainly because of its anti-spasmodic, analgesic (pain-killing) and rubefacient (warming) properties, which find application not only for conditions such as arthritis and rheumatism but also for digestive pain,

menstrual cramp, constipation and related ailments.

Other applications of rosemary, such as its use for hair and skin care, as an insect repellent and as a perfumery ingredient, are considered below under the heading 'Secondary Applications'.

ROSEMARY AS A TONIC

As a **fortifying** and **stimulating** remedy, rosemary has a profound effect on all the systems of the body. According to Rudolf Steiner, the innovative spiritual thinker and founder of the 'Anthroposophy' movement, rosemary is above all a **restorative** remedy which strengthens the vital centre of an individual and increases the activity of the whole metabolism:

> It restores the balance of the calorific body and activates the blood processes (blood is the privileged medium of the heating principle in the human body). It is thus recommended for anaemia, insufficient menstruation, and troubles of blood irrigation. It acts on the liver as well. A better irrigation of the organs eases the action of astral and vital forces and stimulates metabolism ... it promotes the assimilation of sugar (in diabetes) and is indicated to rebuild the nervous system after long, intense intellectual activity.[1]

The **regenerative** effect of rosemary on the central

nervous system is very marked, especially where there
is a reduction in the functioning of the senses, such as
a loss of one's sense of smell, poor eyesight, speech
impairment or temporary paralysis (wasting diseases).
This makes it a valuable remedy for the elderly or during convalescence.

Rosemary has also been called 'the middle-aged
executive's best friend' because it can help to lower
cholesterol levels in the blood while acting as a tonic to
the heart. As a **nervine** and **anti-depressant**, rosemary is indicated for all types of nervous debility
including headaches and migraines resulting from
stress. Valnet recommends rosemary essence especially
for cardiac complaints of nervous origin such as palpitations, as well as for **aphrodisiac** baths! Rosemary
is, however, contra-indicated if blood-pressure is very
high, due to its **hypertensive** effect.

As a **cholagogue** (liver tonic) and **hepatobiliary**
stimulant (increasing the secretion of bile), rosemary is
of benefit in conditions such as cholecystitis, cirrhosis,
gallstones and jaundice. It has also been found to **stimulate the adrenal cortex**, which in turn affects the
metabolic rate of the body and the distribution of fat —
which may be of value in obesity. Rosemary also acts as
a tonic to the reproductive system, and as an **emmenagogue** (promoting menstruation) should be avoided during pregnancy.

ROSEMARY AS A PROPHYLACTIC AGENT

Rosemary has a long history of use as a **prophylactic** (preventative) against infectious illness simply through vaporization. Sprigs of rosemary were burned for their disinfectant properties in French hospitals right up until the end of the last century. As a **pulmonary (lung) antiseptic** it is especially good for the treatment of respiratory conditions such as asthma, bronchitis, colds, sinusitis, whooping cough and flu. Catarrhal conditions respond best to steam inhalations, which clear the head on both the physical and mental plane. As a **diaphoretic** (inducing sweating) rosemary is valuable for infectious conditions involving fever.

Its **bactericidal** properties also make rosemary valuable for the treatment of many common conditions such as boils, spots, bad breath and gum infections. It can also be used as a **disinfectant** for household purposes.

FOR BRINGING WARMTH, MOBILITY AND PAIN RELIEF

Rosemary is well known as the principal ingredient in the famous 'Queen of Hungary Water'. By using this preparation, the 72-year-old Queen of Hungary was apparently transformed from being paralytic and gout-ridden into a revitalized beauty whom the King of Poland subsequently sought to marry! The 'Water' was not, as many imagine, some kind of rejuvenating cosmetic lotion but an excellent **detoxifying** and **regenerative** remedy for the whole system. Rosemary is in fact useful for all types of complaints affecting the bones, joints and muscles because of its specific combination of actions: 'To treat problems that manifest in the bones or muscles effectively, digestion and assimilation have to work well, as do the various aspects of elimination.'[2]

- As a **diuretic** (cleanser), rosemary can aid elimination via the kidneys.
- As an **analgesic** (pain-killing) and **anti-inflammatory** oil, it can help to ease pain and reduce inflammation when applied as a liniment.
- As a **rubefacient** (warming) oil and by **stimulating the circulation** it increases blood flow to the muscles and joints, releasing toxins locally.
- As a **digestive tonic** and **hepatic (liver) remedy** it aids assimilation and digestion, thus preventing the system from becoming congested.
- As a **carminative** and **anti-spasmodic** agent, rosemary can help to alleviate muscle spasms related to the digestive, nervous or reproductive systems, as in cases of dyspepsia, sciatica, neuralgia or dysmenorrhoea.

SECONDARY APPLICATIONS

Rosemary acts as a **stimulant to the hair follicles**, valuable for premature baldness. It is also good for combating dandruff. As an **insecticide** and **vermifuge** it is effective against moths, lice, fleas and garden greenfly (used in a spray).

As a **deodorant** and **astringent**, rosemary oil is used in eau-de-Colognes and some cosmetic lotions.

Rosemary is also used in food products as an **antioxidant,** especially for preserving meats.

CHAPTER SIX

Methods of Use, Safety Data and Storage Precautions

> Seethe much Rosemary, and bathe therein to make thee lusty, lively, joyfull, likeing and youngly.
>
> William Langham, *The Garden of Health* (1579)

METHODS OF USE

Rosemary in the Bath

Add 8–10 drops of rosemary oil to the bath water once the bath is full, then relax in the water for at least 10 minutes. For bathing the feet or hands, add 6–8 drops of rosemary oil to a bowl or shallow bath of warm water and soak for 5–10 minutes.

Compress/Poultice

A simple disinfectant compress can be made by dipping a flannel (face cloth) or piece of cotton wool (cotton ball) in a bowl of water (steaming hot or ice cold, as required) to which has been added 3–5 drops of rosemary oil.

A poultice can be made by adding a few drops of rosemary to a clay or kaolin base, mixing well and applying where necessary.

Culinary Uses

Rosemary is one of the most popular herbs used in cooking, especially for flavouring lamb and poultry dishes. A few drops of rosemary oil may be used for flavouring savoury sauces, but in general it is best to use the herb. Fresh rosemary is available at all times of the year because it is an evergreen – dried rosemary is also very useful since the herb retains its flavour and scent for a long time once dried. For instructions on how to prepare a tisane and for some traditional recipes using rosemary, *see Appendix A*.

Direct / Neat Application

Like most essential oils, rosemary oil should not be used neat on the skin (unless specifically directed).

Gargling and Dental Care

For the treatment of mouth and gum infections, add 3 or 4 drops of rosemary oil to a glass of warm water, mix well, then rinse your mouth and/or gargle with this solution.

Inhalation

Add up to 8 drops of rosemary to a tissue or handkerchief for inhalation throughout the day. Rosemary is best *not* used at night because of its stimulating effect.

For respiratory complaints, make a steam inhalation by adding about 5 drops of rosemary to a bowl of steaming water. Cover your head with a towel and breathe deeply for about 5–10 minutes, keeping your eyes closed.

Massage

Before being applied to the skin for massage purposes, rosemary (like other essential oils) should always be mixed with a light vegetable oil carrier or base such as sweet almond oil, jojoba or grapeseed – although sunflower or soya oil will also suffice. Jojoba oil (being a liquid wax) does not go rancid – otherwise a little wheatgerm oil should be added to the blend to prolong its shelf life. The dilution should be in the region of 2–3 per cent – though sometimes 5 per cent may be used for a concentrated effect, as in the case of treating local muscular pain for example.

As a rough guideline, 20 drops of essential oil equals 1 millilitre, so an easy way of calculating the proportions for general use is to measure the carrier oil in millilitres, then add about half the number of drops of essential oil – this gives a 2.5 per cent dilution:

100 ml base oil	50 drops rosemary essential oil
50 ml base oil	25 drops
1 tbs *(approx. 15 ml base oil)*	7–8 drops
1 tsp *(approx. 5 ml base oil)*	2–3 drops

Shampoo and Hair Care

Buy a good neutral-pH shampoo and add your own rosemary oil to it — rosemary is especially suited to dark hair, giving it shine and body. To a 100-ml bottle add about 60 drops of rosemary oil. An alcohol-based scalp rub can be made by adding 5 ml of rosemary to 100 ml of vodka — this can be used to rid the hair of fleas and lice (though it should not be used on irritated skin). Make a simple hair conditioner by adding a few drops of rosemary oil to the final rinse water.

Sitz Bath / Douche

For vaginal and genito-urinary infections, add 6–8 drops of rosemary oil to a bowl of warm water and bathe the affected area.

Skin Treatments:
Creams, Gels, Lotions, Masks and Oils

The proportions used for mixing skin creams, gels, masks and oils are the same as for massage purposes – see above. For skin care, carrier oils such as avocado, hazelnut, borage, peach and apricot kernel can be included in the blend to suit different skin types.

A light, simple rosemary water can be made up using 100 ml distilled water and 10–15 drops of rosemary oil – shake well before use.

Vaporization

There are many vaporizing methods available now – you can use a terracotta oil burner or an electric diffuser, or you can simply put a few drops of rosemary oil in a small bowl of hot water placed on a radiator or other source of heat. This method is particularly useful for disinfecting a sick room and preventing the spread of contagious illness. Rosemary may also be used to repel insects in this manner.

Other Methods

Many common conditions benefit from combining aromatherapy with other approaches such as herbal medicine, acupuncture, osteopathy, counselling, dietary changes and exercise. Essential oils and allopathic medicines can also complement one another — if in doubt, seek professional advice.

Internal Use

Some medical herbalists in the UK advocate taking essential oils internally for specific purposes, in the form of capsules or pessaries. This is common practice in France, where essential oils are used alongside allopathic medicine by qualified doctors also trained in naturopathy. In Britain, however, where essential oils are employed principally by aromatherapists and by the general public for use in the home, internal consumption is *not* recommended because of the oils' high concentration and the potential damage they can cause to the delicate mucous membranes.

SAFETY DATA

Rosemary oil is non-irritating and non-sensitizing — at up to 10 per cent dilution — to human skin. It is, however, slightly toxic due to its high ketone content — although this depends on the specific type and source of rosemary oil (*see Chapter 4 and Appendix B*). Rosemary oil is contra-indicated in the following cases:

- High blood-pressure: Because it stimulates the circulation, heart and nervous system, rosemary oil

is best avoided by those suffering from high
blood-pressure.

- Epilepsy: 'Rosemary has been implicated in inducing
  epilepsy in people with family trends and there was
  an increase in the incidence of epileptic fits in
  epileptic patients massaged with rosemary oil.'[1]

- Pregnancy: Rosemary oil should be avoided during
  pregnancy because it is an emmenagogue – that is, it
  promotes menstruation.

- Muscular sclerosis: '... Rosemary should never be
  used on Multiple Sclerosis sufferers. She [a herbalist]
  had treated an MS client suffering from painful
  muscular spasm after an aromatherapist had used
  only two drops of Rosemary in a blend for
  massaging the legs. In MS sufferers, the myelin
  sheath surrounding nerves in the brain and spinal
  cord become damaged. When a nerve stimulant
  such as Rosemary was used, it is like sending
  electricity along a bunch of bare wires – all sorts
  of short circuits can happen.'[2]

- Special care should be taken when using essential
  oils for treating babies and young children, because
  of the high concentration levels of the oils. Despite
  rosemary's relatively low toxicity level, it is not
  advisable to use it for treating children under
  5 years of age – and always dilute it to twice the
  recommended proportions before using it for
  children up to 12 years of age. 'Rosemary should ...
  not be used on children: the ketone content is
  neurotoxic.'[3]

Note:

ESSENTIAL OILS SHOULD NOT BE TAKEN INTERNALLY!

STORAGE

For storage purposes rosemary oil should be kept in an air-tight dark glass container, away from light and heat and well out of the reach of children or pets. The pure oil can also interact with certain plastics – plastic containers are therefore best avoided.

IT IS VERY IMPORTANT TO OBTAIN ROSEMARY OIL FROM A REPUTABLE SOURCE TO ENSURE A SAFE AND EFFECTIVE THERAPEUTIC RESULT!

PART II

A–Z of Health & Beauty Applications

amenorrhoea (absent/irregular periods); arteriosclerosis; arthritis; asthma; boil (furuncle)/abscess; bronchitis; bursitis; carbuncles; cellulite; chilblains; colds; colitis; constipation; coughs; dandruff; debility (nervous); depression; disinfectant; dysmenorrhoea (period pain); dyspepsia (indigestion) and flatulence; faintness/dizziness; fever; flu; gout; hair care; hangover; headaches; immune system (to strengthen); insect repellent; jetlag; laryngitis; liver problems/congestion; low blood-pressure (hypotension); lumbago; migraine; mouth and gum infections; muscular aches and pains; neuralgia; oedema (fluid retention); palpitations (tachycardia); perfume; perspiration (excessive); pets/animal care; rheumatism; sciatica; sinusitis; skin care; sore throat; sprains; stress; varicose veins; whooping cough

ACNE (AND SPOTS)
– *see* **Skin Care**

ALOPECIA/BALDNESS
– *see* **Hair Care**

AMENORRHOEA
(ABSENT/IRREGULAR PERIODS)
The absence of menstruation or a scanty or missed period is common at the onset of puberty or during the menopause. However, apart from during pregnancy, a

woman's monthly cycle can become irregular as a result of emotional stress, shock, hormonal imbalance or a serious illness. Girls and women suffering from anorexia nervosa can often stop menstruating due to a lack of nutrients which are needed to synthesize the body's hormones. As a tonic and emmenogogue, rosemary oil can help to regulate and reassert a natural rhythm.

- Gently massage the abdomen with 7–8 drops of rosemary oil in 1 tbs of carrier oil each day, especially in the few days leading up to the onset of menstruation.
- Use a few drops of rosemary oil in the bath regularly, and in a massage or body oil – *see pages 36–7* for preparing massage oils.
- Use rosemary oil in cooking. Avoid stimulants like tea, coffee and alcohol – instead, drink herb teas especially raspberry, yarrow and rose hip.
- Other oils of benefit: rose, yarrow, clary sage, marjoram and myrrh (best used in combination).

Note:

DO NOT USE ROSEMARY OIL DURING PREGNANCY.

See also **Dysmenorrhoea (Period Pain)**

ARTERIOSCLEROSIS
Arteriosclerosis is caused by a slow build-up of fatty deposits in the lining of the coronary arteries leading to

the heart. The arteries become narrower in places, restricting the flow of blood and oxygen to the heart. This can lead to angina, a severe pain in the chest usually brought on by stress or exercise. The danger of arteriosclerosis is that it can result in a heart attack if the warning signs are not heeded in time. Diet needs to be assessed, stress levels reduced, and a more relaxed lifestyle which includes gentle exercise should be taken up. Aromatherapy massage can help to reduce stress and anxiety levels – the use of garlic and rosemary has also been shown to reduce cholesterol levels in the blood while acting as a tonic to the heart. In one case history, a woman suffering from arteriosclerosis, backache and fluid retention was treated regularly with a blend of rosemary, juniper and frankincense as a means of overcoming congestion in the body: 'I worked on her back, wrists, elbows and ankles and she said she felt much better with less aching and more energy. She noticed her urine was strong after the treatment followed by a decrease in fluid retention.'[1]

- Use relaxing oils such as lavender or chamomile for baths, massage and vaporization on a daily basis to reduce stress levels.
- Have a massage at least once a week using 30 drops of rosemary oil in 50 ml of a vegetable carrier oil to improve circulation.
- Take rosemary as a herbal tea and use in cooking; garlic can be taken in the form of capsules.

See also **Stress**

ARTHRITIS

There are several different kinds of arthritis – but all signify the body's inability to eliminate toxic waste efficiently. This causes excess uric acid to be deposited as crystals in the joint spaces. The two most common forms are rheumatoid arthritis, which can affect all age groups, and osteoarthritis, which usually occurs in the elderly. Both are forms of joint distress which can result in pain, inflammation and sometimes deformity. Stress, emotional conflict, lack of exercise and poor diet all contribute to these conditions. Aromatic baths and massage can help eliminate the toxic waste, as well as provide relief from pain. Rosemary, due to its analgesic, stimulating and detoxifying qualities, is one of the most useful remedies for all types of arthritis.

> I applied a cool compress of juniper, lavender and rosemary and wrapped her knee in a towel … The compress was repeated again after 15 minutes, then I massaged her unaffected knee with the same oils. She was delighted with the results which were relief from pain and increased mobility to the joints.[2]

- Make a massage oil by mixing 30 drops of rosemary oil with 50 ml of a vegetable carrier oil. Apply twice daily.
- Add 8–10 drops of rosemary oil to the bath for pain relief.

Note:

THERE ARE SEVERAL OTHER OILS WHICH ARE OF
GREAT BENEFIT IN ARTHRITIS: FOR DETOXIFYING —
CYPRESS, FENNEL, JUNIPER, LEMON AND TEA TREE;
FOR PAIN RELIEF — CHAMOMILE, LAVENDER AND
MARJORAM; FOR STIMULATING GREATER MOBILITY —
PINE, BLACK PEPPER, GINGER.

See also **Gout**, **Muscular Aches and Pains**, **Rheumatism**

ASTHMA

Asthma, characterized by wheezing and shortness of breath, commonly appears during early childhood and often ceases at puberty. It usually runs in families and, like many allergic conditions, can be brought on by a number of different factors including diet, contact with allergens (such as dust, polish, hairspray or feathers), climatic conditions (especially damp), strenuous exercise and/or underlying emotional issues. Many things can be done to alleviate asthma if the cause of the attack and the pattern of the illness can be identified. As a cephalic and anti-spasmodic oil, rosemary (especially combined with massage) is very helpful for asthma. Used as a preventative measure it can keep attacks from occurring so frequently.

- Mix 7 drops of rosemary with 1 tbs sweet almond oil and massage the back in long sweeping movements,

starting at the base of the spine, up over the
shoulders, then down the sides of the body.

- Use rosemary in vaporizers and in the bath at home
  as a general precautionary measure.
- Other oils of benefit: lavender, frankincense,
  geranium, rose, chamomile.

BALDNESS/ALOPECIA
– *see* **Hair Care**

BOIL (FURUNCLE)/ABSCESS
A boil is a localized painful swelling and inflammation
of the skin caused by the infection of a sebaceous gland.
Boils usually appear when the body is run down or
stressed, at times of hormonal upheaval or due to a
blood disorder. Whatever the cause, boils indicate that
the system is in need of purification – avoid stimulants,
eat lots of fresh fruit and vegetables and drink plenty of
water or herb teas (especially those which purify the
blood).

- If the boil/abscess has already formed, apply a warm
  poultice of clay containing 3–4 drops of rosemary
  oil. Leave for half an hour to draw the liquid/pus,
  then bathe gently with water. Alternatively, apply a
  warm flannel (face cloth) which has been soaked in a
  rosemary solution. Repeat two or three times a day.
- If the boil/abscess is severe, cover with a gauze pad
  soaked in rosemary oil for 12 hours. If there is still

no improvement, seek medical advice.
Add 8–10 drops of rosemary oil to the bath as a
general disinfectant measure.

Note:

**TEA TREE OIL AND LAVENDER MAY BE USED
IN THE SAME MANNER.**

See also **Carbuncles**

BRONCHITIS

Bronchitis indicates an inflammation of the bronchial
tubes, accompanied by coughing and mucus congestion. Acute bronchitis usually starts with a cold or sore
throat, which then develops into a fever that lasts a
few days. Chronic bronchitis is a long-term condition,
without fever, which is aggravated by smoking, a damp
climate, air pollution and poor nutrition (especially too
many dairy products). In such conditions rosemary can
be of great benefit by helping to combat the infection,
reduce fever, ease coughing and help the body expel
mucus. It can also help to reinforce the body's immune
mechanism and prevent the infection from spreading.

Note:

**BRONCHITIS CAN LEAD TO COMPLICATIONS,
ESPECIALLY IN THE VERY YOUNG AND ELDERLY —
PROFESSIONAL HELP SHOULD BE SOUGHT
IMMEDIATELY IF THE CONDITION DETERIORATES.**

- At the onset, regular steam inhalations will help to prevent the infection from developing and help to soothe coughing – add 5 drops of rosemary to a bowl of steaming hot water and inhale for 5–10 minutes.
- Hot baths with 8–10 drops of rosemary added encourage sweating, the body's natural response to infection – it also has a similar effect to steam inhalation. When feverish, especially if the temperature is high, keep the bath water cool.
- Massage the chest, back and throat with a 2.5 per cent blend of rosemary in a light base oil or cream – 3 drops to 1 tsp of cream or base oil.
- Use a vaporizer in the home or in the workplace to prevent the spread of infection. A few drops of pure rosemary oil can also be put on a tissue or handkerchief for inhalation throughout the day.
- Other oils of benefit: tea tree, lavender, eucalyptus.

See also **Colds, Coughs, Fever, Flu, Sinusitis, Sore Throat**

BURSITIS
Bursitis is caused by an inflammation of the *bursae*, small water-filled cushions in the elbow ('tennis elbow') or knee joints ('housemaids knee'). The condition may be caused by an accident or hard knock to the joint – or it may show a degenerative rheumatic tendency.
- Make a massage oil by mixing 30 drops of rosemary

oil with 50 ml of a vegetable carrier oil; apply twice daily to the affected area.

See also **Arthritis, Rheumatism**

CARBUNCLES

A collection of boils caused by the *Staphylococcus aureus* bacteria – characterized by a painful node covered with tight red skin that later becomes thick and discharges pus. Commonly found on the upper back, nape of the neck or the buttocks. As a good antiseptic and anti-tox-ic agent, rosemary is a useful oil for this condition.

Keep the area clean – apply a warm rosemary compress to the site of the problem 3 times a day. Add 8–10 drops of rosemary to the bath as a disinfectant measure.

Note:

TEA TREE AND LAVENDER OIL CAN BE USED IN THE SAME MANNER.

See also **Boil (Furuncle)/Abscess**

CELLULITE

A remedy which removes cellulite would be a miracle indeed! This fatty, orange peel-like cell tissue com-monly found on the thighs, legs and upper arms is very stubborn to shift even after considerable weight loss from other parts of the body has been achieved. There are plenty of creams and lotions on the market which claim to help eliminate cellulite, many with dubious results. As a circulatory stimulant and rubefacient oil, rosemary can certainly help to increase the local circulation, bringing warmth to the area and helping to break down congestion within the system. Vigorous massage and the brisk use of a loofah or scrubbing brush in the bath can also help to combat this distressing condition. Correct diet and regular exercise are of course also vitally important.

- Use 8–10 drops of rosemary in the bath.
  Alternatively, if possible, apply a few drops to
  a brush or loofah and rub the affected areas
  briskly while bathing.
- Make up a concentrated massage oil using 10 drops
  of rosemary to 1 tbs base oil and rub the affected
  areas vigorously. (A full body massage also helps to
  enhance circulation generally.)

See also **Skin Care**

CHILBLAINS
Small, painful reddish-blue swellings which are sometimes itchy, mostly occurring on the toes or fingertips, usually as a result of poor circulation or cold. Vitamin and mineral deficiency can also contribute to the problem. Exercise and warm clothing are important preventative measures.

- A regular stimulating massage treatment is beneficial

for bringing warmth to the area. Local blood
circulation can be improved by massaging the feet or
affected area with 2 drops each of rosemary and
black pepper in 1 tsp carrier oil.
- Applying neat tea tree oil (or lemon juice) to the
chilblain can be effective.

COLDS

There are at least 30 different strains of the virus which
can cause the common cold or, in medical terms,
coryza. This highly contagious infection affects the
upper respiratory tract, and the symptoms are well
known: sore throat, coughing, feverishness, aching
limbs, sneezing, fatigue and catarrh. Rosemary oil can
do much to reduce the duration or severity of the
illness and help to prevent secondary infections such
as bronchitis, sinusitis or ear infections.

- Add a few drops to a hankie or to a vaporizer for
inhalation throughout the day.
- Take a daily hot bath adding 8–10 drops of rosemary
to the water – this soothes aching limbs and also acts
as a kind of steam inhalation.
- For a sore throat, add 4–5 drops of rosemary to a
glass of warm water, mix well and gargle. Repeat 2
or 3 times a day at least.
- For a cough, make up a concentrated chest rub by
mixing 5 drops of rosemary with 5 drops of marjoram
(or benzoin) in 1 dessertspoon of carrier oil; apply to
the chest and upper back. Repeat at least twice a day.

the chest and upper back. Repeat at least twice a day.

- As a steam inhalation, add 5–6 drops of rosemary oil
  to a bowl of steaming water, cover your head with
  towel and breathe deeply for 5–10 minutes with your
  eyes closed … very hot steam is in itself a hostile
  environment for viruses. Repeat at least twice a day.
- Other measures: take a course of garlic capsules and
  vitamin C tablets. Use tea tree, lavender or
  eucalyptus in vaporizers throughout the illness;
  marjoram or chamomile oil can also be used in baths
  to soothe aching limbs and encourage restful sleep.

See also **Bronchitis, Coughs, Fever, Flu, Sinusitis, Sore Throat**

COLITIS

Colitis, an inflammation of part of the colon, is the most common complaint affecting the large intestines. Common symptoms include alternating bouts of diarrhoea and constipation, low vitality and sometimes depression. Stress, poor diet and chemical irritants can contribute to the problem.

Rosemary has a natural affinity with the digestive system; as an anti-inflammatory, antiseptic and astringent herb it can help to soothe and heal the lining of the large intestine.

- Mix 7 drops of rosemary with 1 tbs sweet almond oil
  (or another base oil) and massage the abdomen
  gently in a clockwise direction. Repeat twice a day.

CONSTIPATION

Rosemary is good for congested conditions of the body including constipation because of its stimulating effect on the whole system. In one case history a young boy suffering from chronic constipation combined with stress was massaged gently on the abdominal area with a mixture of neroli and rosemary oil:

> The mixture contained 25 drops of neroli plus 2 drops of rosemary in 50 ml of vegetable oil. Rosemary was added because of its general stimulating properties. After this treatment Karl's bowels moved naturally for the first time and although he is still sensitive to stress, with daily massage of this mixture he has continued to have natural bowel movements.[3]

- Mix 7 drops of rosemary with 1 tbs sweet almond oil (or another base oil) and massage the abdomen gently in a clockwise direction. Repeat as required.

COUGHS

Coughing is a natural reflex action aimed at clearing an obstruction or irritation from the respiratory tract. A cough can be dry and unproductive or can be accompanied by mucus discharge, especially when it occurs in association with a cold, flu, bronchitis or other illness.

- Add 5-6 drops of rosemary oil to a bowl of steaming water, cover your head with towel and breathe deeply for 5–10 minutes, keeping your eyes closed. Repeat at least twice a day.

- Make up a concentrated chest rub by mixing 5 drops of rosemary with 5 drops of marjoram (or benzoin) in 1 dessertspoon of carrier oil; apply to the chest and upper back. Repeat at least twice a day.
- Use rosemary (and/or tea-tree, lavender or eucalyptus) in vaporizers throughout the duration of the illness.
- Other measures: keep warm, protect the neck and throat region by wearing a scarf.
- Other oils of benefit: sandalwood, pine, balsam of peru, thyme.

See also **Bronchitis, Colds, Fever, Flu, Sinusitis, Sore Throat**

CRAMP
– *see* **Muscular Aches and Pains**

CUTS AND WOUNDS
– *see* **Disinfectant**

DANDRUFF

This common yet embarrassing problem is caused by *Candida albicans* – a fungus or yeast infection which can affect the scalp. The condition can be further aggravated by overactive sebaceous glands, excessive use of chemical hair preparations, poor diet and stress. Rosemary oil can do much to clear up this problem while at the same time improving the overall condition and health of the hair.

- Mix 25 drops of rosemary oil with 50 ml of slightly warmed jojoba or coconut oil. Massage thoroughly into scalp, wrap your head in warm towels and leave for an hour. Wash out using a 3 per cent rosemary shampoo (about 5 drops of rosemary oil to 1 tsp of a mild shampoo) – apply this mixture first, before the water, otherwise the hair will remain oily. Repeat once a week.
- Use a rosemary shampoo on a daily or regular basis – *see instructions on page 37*.
- A few drops of rosemary oil can be added to the rinse water, conditioning the hair and adding shine.
- Tea tree oil is also very effective for dandruff when used in the same manner.

See also **Hair Care**

DEBILITY (NERVOUS)

Rosemary has been used for centuries as a nerve tonic in cases of debility or nervous exhaustion – and is still specified in the *British Herbal Pharmacopoeia* for 'depressive states with general debility'. It not only stimulates the whole system but also fortifies it – Dr Valnet recommended rosemary in 'fortifying morning baths', especially for children (over 5 years of age) and for general fatigue.

- Add 5–10 drops to the bath or footbath as a reviving 'pick-me-up'.
- Use in baths, massage and inhalations to strengthen the nervous system on a daily basis.

See also **Depression**

DEPRESSION

Depression can take many forms: it is often associated with a lack of energy and listlessness, but can also be accompanied by restlessness or agitation – sufferers sometimes alternating between the two. Rosemary has long been used to help alleviate depression due to its stimulating and uplifting effects. A tonic to the heart and circulation, rosemary is particularly useful for depression related to stressful situations which leave the body listless and lacking in vitality.

- Add 10 drops of rosemary oil to the bath – best used in combination with other anti-depressant oils such as bergamot, lavender and/or jasmine.
- Receiving a regular professional massage using a blend of anti-depressant oils including rosemary can help to encourage feelings of self-worth and well-being. Research has shown that the 'synergistic' combination of smell and touch can have a profoundly nourishing and comforting effect on the psyche.
- For an uplifting/refreshing room fragrance, use rosemary oil in a vaporizer; or add a few drops to a

hankie for use throughout the day.
- Other measures: yoga, meditation and psychotherapy/counselling.
- Other oils of benefit: bergamot, neroli, jasmine, melissa, rose, lavender.

DISINFECTANT

Rosemary has excellent antiseptic properties, and as such it can be used very effectively as a disinfectant for first-aid purposes as well as for more general household chores. It has been used traditionally for cleaning floors: when King James I visited the Bodleian Library in Oxford in the seventeenth century, the floors had been rubbed with the fresh herb. A dilute water solution can be used for swabbing down washable surfaces, and a few drops added to the laundry water will disinfect nappies, clothes, towels, etc., leaving a fresh, clean scent. The vaporized oil can also be used very effectively to disinfect rooms at home or in the workplace, especially during or following infectious illness. It was used in France in this manner until the late nineteenth century.

- Disinfecting clothes, nappies, etc.: for hand washing, add up to 25 drops of rosemary oil to half a litre of warm water; otherwise add up to 50 drops to a liquid detergent before putting into the washing machine.
- For washing floors, surfaces, etc.: add up to 50 drops to a bucket or bowl of water. Stir well before

mopping or wiping surfaces.
- For cleaning small cuts or wounds, etc.: add a few
  drops of neat rosemary to a small bowl of cooled
  boiled water (do not use the oil neat), then swab the
  damaged area using a cotton wool pad.
- Disinfecting sickrooms, bathrooms, workplaces,
  etc.: diffuse rosemary into the air using a vaporizer.

DIZZINESS
— *see* **Faintness/Dizziness**

DYSMENORRHOEA (PERIOD PAIN)
Caused by uterine spasm during menstruation, the fre-
quency and severity of period pain are often also associated with diet and underlying emotional factors. The
excellent analgesic and anti-spasmodic properties of
rosemary make it an excellent remedy for period pains
(best used in combination with the other oils mentioned below).

- Gently massage the abdomen and lower back with
  7 drops of rosemary in 1 tbs carrier oil.
- Hot compresses using a few drops of rosemary on a
  flannel (or on a cloth wrapped round a hot water
  bottle) which is then placed on the abdomen can
  help to relieve the pain.
- Relaxing in a hot rosemary bath eases pain and also
  soothes away stress and tension.
- Other oils of benefit: chamomile, clary sage,
  lavender, rose, marjoram (best used in combination).

DYSPEPSIA (INDIGESTION) AND FLATULENCE

Dyspepsia or indigestion is a common complaint, both among children and adults. As a carminative and anti-spasmodic agent, rosemary is especially valuable for all types of digestive disorders (including flatulence) where there is a strong nervous or emotional element involved. In the *British Herbal Pharmacopoeia* rosemary is indicated for: 'flatulent dyspepsia associated with psychogenic tension'.[4]

- Mix 3 drops of rosemary in 1 tsp of carrier oil and massage the tummy gently in a clockwise direction.
- Other oils of benefit: chamomile, lavender or peppermint oil (used in combination); chamomile, peppermint or fennel tea, with a little honey.

See also **Stress**

FAINTNESS/DIZZINESS

Faintness or dizziness can result from a number of causes: severe shock, sunstroke, hangover, nervous exhaustion or very low blood-pressure. It is also common during the menopause and can be a symptom of pre-menstrual tension (PMT). Rosemary has a revitalizing effect on the mind and body.

- Simply smelling rosemary oil can revive the spirits, helpful in cases of emotional shock, nervous exhaustion, sunstroke, etc.

• Add up to 10 drops of rosemary to the bath as a reviving 'pick-me-up' and to restore equilibrium.

See also **Hangover**

FATIGUE
– *see* **Debility (Nervous)**

FEVER

A raised temperature is a vital and healthy response to infection because it speeds up the body's metabolic rate and strengthens its natural defence systems. In many instances a fever should be allowed to run its course – a process that often culminates in a period of profuse sweating which eventually subsides together with a lowering of the fever. Rosemary oil is a very useful aid for feverish conditions involving infection due to its powerful antiviral, bactericidal and immuno-stimulant qualities. Rosemary oil can also help to induce perspiration when the body needs to 'sweat it out', due to its diaphoretic properties (although it does not cause sweating when the body is in a normal state).

Note:

IF THE FEVER REMAINS HIGH, OR RISES
TO A DANGEROUS LEVEL, SEEK PROFESSIONAL
MEDICAL ADVICE IMMEDIATELY.

• Use rosemary in vaporizers throughout the duration of the illness, but especially at the onset. In addition,

add a few drops to a hankie or pillowcase for
inhalation throughout the day.

Note:

**ROSEMARY IS BEST AVOIDED FOR NIGHT USE
BECAUSE IT CAN CAUSE SLEEPLESSNESS.**

- To help control a high temperature, immerse the
  whole body in a tepid bath containing 3–10 drops
  (depending on the age of the patient) of rosemary oil.
- If the person is too weak to get into a bath, sponge the
  body down using a flannel soaked in tepid water to
  which a few drops of rosemary oil have been added.
- Other measures: drink plenty of pure water or liquids
  to detoxify the system and prevent dehydration.
- Other oils of benefit: peppermint, tea tree,
  eucalyptus, bergamot, lavender.

See also **Bronchitis, Colds, Coughs, Flu, Sinusitis,
Sore Throat**

FLATULENCE
– see **Dyspepsia**

FLU
Influenza is the most common single cause of fever,
although the term is often used to include various un-
identified viral infections characterized by a raised temperature, aching limbs, fatigue, a sore throat and other
respiratory symptoms such as catarrh or a dry cough.

Self-help using essential oils can help to prevent an attack of flu, or at least to reduce the severity of the illness.

- Use rosemary in vaporizers throughout the duration of the illness, but especially at the onset – this may prevent it from developing fully. In addition, add a few drops to a hankie or pillowcase for inhalation throughout the day.
- At the very first sign of infection take a hot bath, adding 8–10 drops of rosemary to the water. Repeat each morning, or every other morning – this is often enough to avert a full-blown attack.
- For a sore throat, add 4–5 drops of rosemary to a glass of warm water, mix well and gargle. Repeat at least 2 or 3 times a day.
- For a cough, make up a concentrated chest rub by mixing 5 drops of rosemary with 5 drops of marjoram (or benzoin) in 1 dessertspoon of carrier oil. Apply to the chest and upper back. Repeat at least twice a day.
- To relieve congestion, add 5–6 drops of rosemary oil to a bowl of steaming water, cover your head with towel and breathe deeply for 5–10 minutes with your eyes closed. Very hot steam is in itself a hostile environment for viruses. Repeat at least twice a day.
- Other measures: take a course of garlic capsules. Tea tree oil is also a very effective prophylactic agent for infections, when used in the same manner as rosemary. Lavender, marjoram or chamomile oil can also be used in baths to soothe aching limbs and encourage restful sleep.

See also **Bronchitis, Colds, Coughs, Fever, Sinusitis, Sore Throat**

GINGIVITIS
— *see* **Mouth and Gum Infections**

GOUT

Gout is a specific kind of joint inflammation caused by a build-up of uric acid in the body. It can be extremely painful. Usually caused by an over-indulgence in rich foods and alcohol, whereby the kidneys cannot successfully eliminate accumulated toxins. Gout usually affects the joints of the toes, but also sometimes those of the fingers. Stress, emotional conflict and lack of exercise all contribute to this condition. Aromatic baths and massage can help eliminate the toxic waste, as well as provide relief from pain. Rosemary, due to its analgesic, stimulating and detoxifying qualities, is one of the most useful remedies for gout.

- Make a massage oil by mixing 30 drops of rosemary oil with 50 ml of a vegetable carrier oil. Apply twice daily.
- Add 8–10 drops of rosemary oil to the bath for pain relief.

Note:

THERE ARE SEVERAL OTHER OILS WHICH ARE OF GREAT BENEFIT IN GOUT: FOR DETOXIFYING — CYPRESS, FENNEL, JUNIPER, LEMON, TEA TREE;

FOR PAIN RELIEF — CHAMOMILE, LAVENDER,
MARJORAM; FOR STIMULATING GREATER MOBILITY —
PINE, BLACK PEPPER, GINGER.

See also **Arthritis**

HAIR CARE

Rosemary oil makes an excellent conditioning treatment for the hair due to its fresh scent, gentle action
and powerful antiseptic properties. It helps to regulate
the activity of the sebaceous glands, cleanses the scalp
of bacterial and fungal infection, and helps to disperse
dead skin cells. By making the hair more healthy and
manageable, rosemary oil benefits all hair types including dry hair, greasy hair, itchy scalp conditions and dandruff. Rosemary also acts as a stimulant to the hair
follicles, making this oil most effective for premature
baldness. It makes the hair shine and is especially recommended for dark hair.

- Choose a mild or pH-neutral shampoo which does
  not strip the hair of its protective acid mantle, then
  add between 1 and 2 per cent of rosemary oil (about
  20–50 drops per 100 ml of mild shampoo —
  alternatively you could use 2–3 drops of tea tree oil
  to one teaspoon of shampoo). Shampoo daily or
  according to your usual routine — this treatment is
  good for all hair types.
- Rosemary oil can also be added to a conditioning

lotion in the same manner (2 per cent), or a few drops put in the final rinse water.

- Hair conditioner: mix 25 drops of rosemary oil with 50 ml of slightly warmed jojoba or coconut oil; massage thoroughly into scalp. Wrap in warm towels and leave for an hour. Wash out using rosemary shampoo – apply the shampoo first, before the water, otherwise the hair will remain oily. Repeat once a week. Tea tree oil can also be used to condition the hair in the same manner.

- A good final rinse for all hair types is to add 5 drops of rosemary and 1 tbs of cider vinegar to the final rinse water. This will help to remove detergent residue and restore the acid equilibrium of the scalp.

See also **Dandruff**

HALITOSIS (BAD BREATH)
– see **Mouth and Gum Infections**

HANGOVER
As a cephalic, stimulating and anti-spasmodic remedy, rosemary oil can help lift the spirits and ease headaches or faintness.

- Add 10 drops of rosemary to the bath water for a deliciously uplifting morning bath. Afterwards, splash on a liberal amount of rosemary eau-de-Cologne – *see* **Perfume**.

See also **Headaches, Faintness/Dizziness**

HEADACHES

Headaches can be caused by a number of different factors: sinus congestion, nervous stress, eye strain, too much sun or too much alcohol! Rosemary oil is especially good for nervous headaches and those associated with congestion due to a cold or sinusitis.

- Inhale rosemary oil from a tissue, or if the head is congested a steam inhalation is generally more effective.
- Headaches brought on by tension or stress can also be eased by a firm neck and shoulder massage using 3 drops of rosemary in 1 tsp carrier oil.
- Lavender oil is also valuable for nervous headaches.

See also **Colds, Hangover, Migraine, Sinusitis, Stress**

HEPATIC DISORDERS
– *see* **Liver Problems/Congestion**

HYPOTENSION
– *see* **Low Blood-pressure**

IMMUNE SYSTEM (TO STRENGTHEN)

The immune response is orchestrated by three distinct groups of cells: the phagocytes, the 'T' cells, and the 'B' cells. These all originate from white blood cells in the bone marrow and serve to protect the body from infection. If this defensive barrier is damaged for some reason, the body becomes vulnerable to invasion by all sorts of pathogenic organisms. The immune system is supported by and closely related to other body functions, especially the lymphatic and nervous systems. Recent research tends to suggest that emotional and psychological factors play a vital role in the efficiency of the immune response. This may help to account for the fact that viral infections and suppressed immune systems are becoming an increasing problem today – while diseases such as Acquired Immune Deficiency Syndrome (AIDS), Chronic Fatigue Syndrome and other viral infections are presenting symptoms not previously encountered. Many essential oils, including rosemary, are very beneficial used in this context since they can assist the body in resisting as well as combating infection:

1 by directly opposing the threatening micro-organisms
2 by stimulating and increasing the activity of the organs and cells involved
3 by building up resistance and promoting the immune system as a whole.

People who use essential oils all the time, as part of their daily bathing, skincare and household routines, mostly have a high level of resistance to illness, 'catching' fewer colds, etc. than average and recovering quickly if they do.[5]

- To help build up resistance levels, take a bath at least twice a week using 8–10 drops of rosemary oil in the water.
- To strengthen the immune system, have a massage once a week using a 2.5 per cent rosemary oil blend – *see instructions on pages 36–7.* If this is not possible, make up a 5 per cent concentrated massage oil blend and rub this firmly into the palms of your hands and soles of your feet once a day.
- Use rosemary and other essential oils as room fragrances on an everyday basis.

Note:

TEA TREE OIL IS THE MOST EFFECTIVE IMMUNO-STIMULANT OIL TO USE IN THIS WAY.

- Other measures: a course of garlic capsules, vitamin E and vitamin C are also indicated.

INDIGESTION
– *see* **Dyspepsia**

INSECT REPELLENT
Rosemary has been used for centuries to repel moths, fleas and other insects. Chests made from rosemary wood were once used to store linen and other cloth in order to preserve them.

- As a preventative measure, rosemary oil can be applied neat to clothing, linen, etc., or a sachet of

the dried herb can be placed in the drawer or
cupboard.

- To keep insects out of the house, apply rosemary to
hanging ribbons around the house, or use a
vaporizer.
- Other measures: there are several other oils with
insect-repellent properties, the most useful being
lavender, citronella, lemongrass, eucalyptus, tea
tree or atlas cedarwood – or a combination of these.

JETLAG

As a fortifying and stimulating oil, rosemary can be
very helpful for those making international journeys
who find themselves exhausted not only by long hours
of travelling but also by jetlag – caused by the crossing
of time zones.

- Add 10 drops of rosemary to the bath as a pick-me-
up – not to be used just before bed.
- Apply a few drops of rosemary to a tissue or
handkerchief for use throughout the trip.
- Other measures: lavender oil is particularly
recommended for jetlag due to its relaxant and
regulating effects.

LARYNGITIS

Laryngitis is characterized by a sore throat, hoarseness
or a temporary loss of voice brought on by an infection,
such as bronchitis or flu, or due to over-straining the
vocal chords.

- Add 4–5 drops of rosemary to a glass of warm
  water, mix well and gargle. Repeat at least 2 or 3
  times a day.
- For a dry cough, make up a concentrated chest rub
  by mixing 5 drops of rosemary with 5 drops of
  sandalwood in 1 dessertspoon of carrier oil. Apply
  to the chest and throat at least twice a day.
- Other oils of benefit: tea tree, lavender, eucalyptus,
  benzoin.

See also **Bronchitis, Coughs, Flu, Sore Throat**

LIVER PROBLEMS/CONGESTION

There are many complaints relating to liver congestion,
inflammation or weakness – notably hepatitis in its various forms (hepatitis A, B, C, D and E). There are many
hepatic oils that can be used to cleanse, detoxify and in
some cases stimulate the liver, but such treatment should
only be offered alongside conventional drug therapy
where severe damage is suspected. Rosemary is one of
the most useful oils for the liver, since it exhibits the
following properties: 'antiviral, stimulant, chologogue;
choleretic: aids excretion of bile by liver, so there is
greater flow of bile; stimulant of adrenal cortex'.[6]

Note:

LIVER AND PANCREATIC DISORDERS CALL FOR A
PROFESSIONAL DIAGNOSIS BEFORE ANY COURSE OF
AROMATHERAPY TREATMENT IS EMBARKED UPON.

- Add 8—10 drops of rosemary to the bath water on a regular basis.
- If there is pain in the liver area, a low dilution of oil (0.25 per cent) can be applied to areas such as the nape of the neck, solar plexus or soles of the feet.
- It is beneficial to use the herb in cooking.

LOW BLOOD-PRESSURE (HYPOTENSION)

Although this condition is less common and has less potential dangers than high blood-pressure (hypertension), it is often accompanied by debilitating symptoms such as dizziness, constant feelings of tiredness and sensitivity to the cold. As a tonic, reviving and stimulating oil, rosemary can help to normalize the blood-pressure by increasing the flow of circulation and bringing a sense of warmth and vigour to the body. Brisk massage is particularly useful to stimulate the entire system, as is gentle exercise taken on a regular basis.

- Make a massage oil by mixing 30 drops of rosemary oil with 50 ml of a vegetable carrier oil. Apply briskly to the entire body, paying particular attention to the extremities (hands and feet).
- Add 8—10 drops of rosemary oil to the bath water on a regular basis.
- Use rosemary oil in a vaporizer at home or in the workplace to uplift the mind and invigorate the body.
- Other oils of benefit: black pepper, ginger, cardamom, pimento.

Note:

**SOME SPICY OILS ARE IRRITATING TO THE
SKIN — USE IN LOW DILUTIONS ONLY.**

See also **Chilblains**

LUMBAGO

Lumbago is a general name for pain in the lower back.
It can have a variety of causes including rheumatism,
arthritis, muscular strain, or kidney or reproductive
problems. The root of the complaint should be identified and treated accordingly, but in many cases the
application of warming, stimulating remedies or hot
compresses can be very helpful. As an analgesic (pain-
killing), rubefacient (warming) and diuretic (cleansing)
oil, rosemary is especially valuable where there is pain,
swelling or lack of mobility.

In one case history, a man suffering from severe
backpain and spasm caused by spondylosis of the spine
turned to aromatherapy as an alternative to conventional pain-killers. A blend containing 10 drops of rosemary, 6 drops of juniper, 5 drops of lavender and 4
drops of bergamot in 50 ml carrier oil was massaged
regularly into his spine, with a full body massage once a
month to help lymph drainage:

> I wanted a powerful, natural analgesic, an anti-depressant
> and something to aid elimination ... This blend has a pro-
> nounced analgesic quality which lasts up to 24 hours. It is
> also sedative and anti-depressant, which helps to break

the circle of pain, muscular spasm and restless nights.

As a result this man was able to reduce his daily intake of pain-killing drugs, and reserve his orthopaedic collar for only the 'bad days'. In addition:

> My physical stature and mobility are greatly improved …
> The most noticeable effect after treatment has been the
> state of mental and physical relaxation and the change
> from negative to positive attitude. I have also become
> more resistant to colds and flu and my body feels more
> alive. Although I am not completely pain free I can plan
> things long term.[7]

- To relieve muscular spasm or if a particular area is very tight or painful, massage with a 5 per cent rosemary oil blend or apply a hot compress (cold if there is inflammation) to which a few drops of rosemary oil have been added.
- Make a massage oil by mixing 30 drops of rosemary oil with 50 ml of a vegetable carrier oil. Apply gently to the affected area.
- Add 8–10 drops of rosemary oil to the bath water on a regular basis.
- There are several oils which are useful for lumbago depending on the cause of the problem, including lavender and chamomile (to ease inflammation and as sedatives), juniper (as a diuretic), and bergamot and geranium (to uplift and regulate the system).

See also **Arthritis, Gout, Muscular Aches and Pains, Rheumatism**

MIGRAINE
Migraine is most commonly a food-related complaint, but an attack can also be triggered by an increase in stress or anxiety. Although aromatherapy is best used as a preventive measure by promoting relaxation as part of your everyday lifestyle, rosemary can also ease the pain and severity of an attack.

For treatment, *see* **Headaches**

MOUTH AND GUM INFECTIONS
There are several types of mouth and gum infections, having different causes. Rosemary, because of its bactericidal (germ-killing) properties, can help to keep the mouth fresh and clean, especially in the following cases:

a   Mouth ulcers – tiny blisters which then burst to form ulcers (2–10 mm in diameter) occurring on the tongue, floor of the mouth or on the inside of the cheeks.

b   Gingivitis – a red spongy swelling of the gums, which bleed easily, especially when cleaning the teeth.

c   Halitosis (bad breath) – caused by poor dental hygiene or by an infection in the body, and aggravated by smoking and dietary factors.

• For mouth ulcers, dilute rosemary to 50 per cent in water, mix well and apply to the spots or ulcers with a cotton bud (cotton swab) – repeat twice daily for 3 days.

- For the treatment of gingivitis and bad breath (halitosis) or other mouth and gum infections, add 3 or 4 drops of rosemary oil to a glass of warm water, mix well, then rinse the mouth and/or gargle on a daily or twice-daily basis. Repeat morning and evening, after brushing the teeth.
- Tea tree oil is also very effective for mouth and gum infections; use as indicated here for rosemary.

MOUTH ULCERS
– *see* **Mouth and Gum Infections**

MUSCULAR ACHES AND PAINS

Muscular aches and pains are a common affliction, caused either by physical over-exertion or by psychological stress and strain. Many people, for example, carry tension in their necks and shoulders, which over a period of time causes the muscles to become tight and painful. The stimulating, penetrating and mild analgesic properties of rosemary make it an excellent remedy for all types of muscular complaints, especially where there is pain or stiffness.

> … a very good oil to use for tired, stiff and overworked muscles. I have used it very successfully in treating athletes, particularly long-distance runners, using rosemary in combination with other oils before training or competitive events, and lavender, usually combined with

marjoram, for massage after training or competing."

- Soaking in a hot bath is an easy and effective way of relaxing the muscles and bringing instant pain relief: 8–10 drops of rosemary oil added to the water will increase the benefits further due to the oil's analgesic (pain-killing) and penetrating qualities.
- Muscular aches and pains respond well to local massage – add about 9 drops of rosemary to 1 tbs of carrier oil and rub into the affected area.
- To relieve muscular spasm or if a particular area is very tight, massage with neat rosemary oil or apply a hot compress to which a few drops of rosemary oil have been added.
- A few drops of rosemary rubbed into the muscles before and immediately after strenuous exercise can help prevent muscular aches and pains from developing.
- Other oils of benefit: lavender, tea tree, marjoram.

See also **Lumbago**, **Neuralgia**, **Sciatica**

NERVOUS EXHAUSTION
– *see* **Debility (Nervous)**

NEURALGIA
Neuralgia (nerve pain) can take many forms – sometimes running the whole length of a nerve, at other times affecting a localized point on the skin's surface. This distressing condition can result from a number of

different causes – an infection, an accident, an osteo-pathic problem or, more commonly, through general debility, poor diet, lack of exercise and stress. As a nerve tonic and pain-killer, rosemary can help over-come neuralgia – but it is vital also to tackle the root of the problem, which may necessitate changes in lifestyle and diet – to include plenty of green vegetables, fruit, oats and a course of vitamin B complex.

- Soaking in a hot bath is an easy and effective way of bringing pain relief: 8–10 drops of rosemary oil added to the water will increase the benefits further due to the oil's analgesic (pain-killing) and penetrat-ing qualities.
- Add about 25–30 drops of rosemary to 50 ml of carrier oil and rub gently into the affected area.
- Other oils of benefit: lavender, peppermint, marjoram (used in combination in the same manner as above); St John's Wort (an infused oil or base oil).

See also **Sciatica**

OEDEMA (FLUID RETENTION)

Oedema is a common complaint, especially during pregnancy and in the overweight. In one case history, a hospital patient suffering from congestive heart failure and severe oedema of the ankles, legs and abdomen was massaged with a blend of rosemary, lavender and frankincense. An area of tight shiny skin on the legs was avoided, however, as this could have increased the flow

of blood back from the veins to the heart, adding strain
to an already over-burdened heart.

> I began using rosemary for its diuretic properties, to help
> reduce oedema ... Over the next few months with con-
> tinued treatment and an increase in her medication, she
> began to lose some of her retained fluid and her ankle and
> leg oedema reduced. As this happened her skin, which
> had been stretched by oedema, became dry and wrin-
> kled. Once the oedema had subsided, the area was
> rubbed with a mixture of sandalwood and sweet almond
> oil to help normalize the texture of the skin.'

- Add about 9 drops of rosemary to 1 tbs of carrier oil
  and rub gently into the affected area.

Note:

ROSEMARY SHOULD NOT BE USED DURING PREGNANCY.

PALPITATIONS (TACHYCARDIA)

This is a general term used to describe an irregular
heartbeat – either 'missing a beat' or a rapid 'fluttering'
of the heart. It can be brought on by exercise but is
usually associated with high blood-pressure or stress. It
is particularly common during the menopause.

- Inhalations of rosemary can help regulate a rapidly
  beating heart, although ylang ylang is recognized as
  the most useful oil for palpitations.
- Regular aromatic bathing and massage, using

(individually or in combination) ylang ylang, lavender, neroli, rose or chamomile also helps to reduce stress levels and anxiety, which often trigger tachycardia.

See also **Stress**

PERIOD PAIN
– see **Dysmenorrhoea**

PERFUME

Rosemary has been used for hundreds of years to perfume linen, paper, leather, pot pourris and many other household items, including wood. Applied neat it does not leave a greasy mark, yet the strong scent repels moths and lasts for a long time. It was also used for perfuming ink! However, the most traditional way of using rosemary as a perfume is in the form of an eau-de-Cologne, or blended toilet-water. 'Queen of Hungary Water' was originally prepared by infusing freshly picked rosemary flowers in wine for use as a body tonic rub – but it was subsequently revised and reformulated as a cosmetic preparation or rosemary 'eau-de-Cologne'. A modern version of the perfume called 'Hungary Water' runs as follows:

1 ml (20 drops) rosemary oil	0.5 ml (10 drops) peppermint oil
3 ml (60 drops) verbena oil	50 ml rosewater
1 ml (20 drops) orange oil	50 ml orange flower water

0.5 ml (10 drops) lime oil   400 ml alcohol
                                    (vodka)

PERSPIRATION (EXCESSIVE)
Rosemary can be used as an excellent disinfectant and
deodorant, having a fresh, pleasing scent.

- Add 5–10 drops of rosemary oil to a bowl of warm
  water and soak the feet nightly for 5 minutes.
- Splash rosemary eau-de-Cologne (*see* **Perfume**)
  beneath the arms (or on other areas prone to
  excessive perspiration) in the morning/evening
  after bathing.
- Use rosemary in the bath on a regular basis – but not
  just before retiring for the night, as it can prevent
  sleep.

PETS/ANIMAL CARE
Essential oils are being increasingly employed for the
treatment of common ailments in veterinary practice
and for the care of domestic pets – particularly dogs,
cats and horses.

- Fleas – use rosemary shampoo (*see instructions page
  37*) on a daily basis – leave for 3–5 minutes before
  washing out. Afterwards, or between washes, wipe
  the coat with a moist sponge sprinkled with 10–20
  drops of pure rosemary oil. This also improves the
  condition of the coat.

RHEUMATISM

The term 'rheumatism' is used medically to describe a whole range of disorders which involve pain in the muscles or joints, including the various forms of arthritis and gout. Generally speaking, however, rheumatism refers specifically to muscular pain, whereas arthritis and gout are associated with pain located within the joints themselves. Rosemary can help to ease rheumatic pain due to its analgesic (pain-killing) qualities – it also increases local blood circulation and enhances mobility. Since rheumatism, like arthritis, is aggravated by an accumulation of toxins in the system, the diet and lifestyle should be assessed to try to get at the root of the problem.

- Massage is itself very helpful for rheumatic pains because it stimulates the circulation and helps to remove toxins. Make up a concentrated massage oil by mixing 30 drops of rosemary oil with 50 ml of a vegetable carrier oil. Apply twice daily.
- Add 8–10 drops of rosemary oil to the bath water for pain relief.
- Other oils of benefit: chamomile, tea tree, lavender, marjoram.

See also **Arthritis, Gout, Muscular Aches and Pains**

SCIATICA

This distressing condition is a form or neuralgia (nerve

pain) characterized by an intense shooting pain or tenderness felt along the length of the sciatic nerve, which runs from the back of the thigh to the lower calf. The term is also often used to describe nerve pain which radiates from the lower back to the thigh. There may be a misalignment of the hips or lower spine which causes pressure to the sciatic nerve, but the cause of the problem often lies in abdominal congestion and constipation. As a nerve tonic, analgesic and anti-spasmodic, rosemary can be of great relief to those suffering from sciatica — it also acts as a stimulant for the whole system, including the abdominal region, thus helping to relieve any congestion in this area. Exercise, lifestyle and diet should also be assessed. 'Where there is neuralgia or nerve pain, relaxing nervines and tonics will help ... massage of the lower back and legs may help a lot.'[10]

- Gentle massage is itself very helpful for sciatica, as indicated above. Make up a concentrated massage oil by mixing 30 drops of rosemary oil with 50 ml of a vegetable carrier oil. Apply twice daily.
- Add 8–10 drops of rosemary oil to the bath water for pain relief.
- Other oils of benefit: peppermint, lavender, marjoram (use in combination); also the infused or base oil St John's Wort.

See also **Neuralgia**

SINUSITIS

Sinusitis is an infection of the mucous membranes lining the bony cavities behind, above and on each side of the nose. It usually follows a cold, hayfever or prolonged exposure to chilly, damp air. An acute attack is often accompanied by congested headaches and catarrh, sometimes with fever. Chronic or long-term sinusitis indicates a mild infection which causes the nose to be continually blocked and a dull pain or feeling of tension to manifest in the area between the eyes. People who suffer from constant or repeated attacks of sinusitis often suffer from allergies – especially to gluten and cow's milk.

Note:

SINUSITIS CAN LEAD TO SECONDARY INFECTIONS, NOTABLY EAR INFECTIONS AND VERY OCCASIONALLY MENINGITIS – IF WORRIED, SEEK PROFESSIONAL MEDICAL ADVICE IMMEDIATELY.

- Steam inhalations relieve congestion and fight infection – use 5 drops of rosemary oil in a bowl of steaming water, cover your head with a towel and inhale deeply for 5–10 minutes, keeping your eyes closed. Repeat several times a day.
- Use 8–10 drops in the bath water – this acts as a kind of steam inhalation.
- Use rosemary oil in a vaporizer – or put a few drops onto your pillow or on a hankie for use throughout the day.

- Other measures: A course of garlic capsules
  is indicated. Certain foods, especially dairy
  produce (made from cow's milk) and wheat
  products aggravate the problem, and should be
  eliminated from the diet as much as possible
  during treatment.
- Other oils of benefit: eucalyptus, tea tree,
  peppermint.

See also **Colds, Fever, Flu, Headaches**

SKIN CARE

The condition of the skin expresses the overall health of
the person. A relaxed attitude, together with a well-
balanced diet, enough exercise and a daily intake of
plenty of spring water or herb teas, all help to keep the
system in top condition. A stressful lifestyle, on the
other hand, and too much coffee, tea and alcohol all
take their toll on the skin, which soon starts to look
dull and lifeless.

The appearance of the skin also depends on the
type of skin care routine adopted. Products containing mineral oil or lanolin are not absorbed into the
lower dermal layers where the newly emerging cells
require optimum nourishment. Alcohol-based products dehydrate the skin and can cause irritation, as can
many other synthetic ingredients. In contrast, natural
vegetable oils, waxes and creams, together with spe-
cially selected essential oils, are ideal cosmetic aids
because they are *highly* penetrative and can reach the

small blood capillaries in the deeper dermal layers, thus rejuvenating the skin 'from within'.

Rosemary is one of the ancient herbs renowned for its revitalizing and youth-giving qualities. Is there any truth in this claim – or is it no more than just an old wives' tale?

> The research started by looking for anti-oxidant properties among herbs which had a tradition for prolonging life or reducing ageing – plants like sage and rosemary. Indeed, herb enthusiasts will not be surprised to discover that these old favourites do have very potent anti-oxidant properties indeed.

And now for the bad news...

> The chemicals concerned are non-volatile [and destroyed by heat] so are not in the essential oils from either plant ... among the first to be identified is rosmaric acid from rosemary which is eight times more effective as an anti-oxidant than many of the synthetic food preservatives like butylated hydroxytoluene and butylated hydroxyanisole.[11]

Anti-oxidants, apart from their application for the preservation of food – another one of rosemary's valuable assets – are also extremely beneficial for preserving a youthful complexion. Nevertheless, since the chemicals concerned are not present in the essential oil, in order to gain the full benefits the whole herb should be utilized. An old recipe for making a 'Rejuvenating

Lotion' (a variation on the 'Queen of Hungary Water')
runs as follows:

  1 tbs fresh rosemary
  1 tbs fresh mint
  60 ml witch-hazel
  120 ml rosewater
  Grated peel of a quarter of one orange and a quarter
  of one lemon.
  Mix all together, pour into a bottle and steep for a
  week. Strain before using.[12]

Rosemary is also a valuable skin care agent because,
although it has excellent antiseptic properties, it is also
an effective deodorant and astringent. It can help combat greasy skin and spots used in combination with
other oils such as lavender or tea tree, and helps to regulate the production of seborrhea. However, because
rosemary is also renowned as a powerful stimulant of
the hair follicles, it is best for women not to apply copi-
ous amounts to the face (lest you find yourself turning
into the bearded lady!)

• As a cleanser/toner for congested skin, blend 10
  drops each of rosemary, tea tree and lavender
  essential oils with 25 ml of witch-hazel and 75 ml
  distilled water (or another flower water). Apply
  morning and night before moisturizing the skin.
• Add 8–10 drops of rosemary oil to the bath water
  – this also acts as a facial steam.

- Have a facial sauna at least once a week using 3–5
  drops of rosemary – *see page 36*.

Note:

**TEA TREE OIL OR LAVENDER MAY BE
USED IN THE SAME MANNER.**

SORE THROAT

A sore throat often accompanies other respiratory
infections such as flu, bronchitis and the common cold.
It is often the first sign of illness, and if treated immediately can prevent further infection from developing –
or at least shorten the duration of the disease.

- Add 3 or 4 drops of rosemary oil to a glass of warm
  water, mix well, and gargle at least two or three times
  a day. Continue until the condition has cleared up.
- Other oils of benefit: tea tree, sage, thyme.

See also **Bronchitis, Colds, Flu, Laryngitis**

SPRAINS

Pulled muscles or sprained ligaments or tendons
respond well to treatment with essential oils. As an
analgesic (pain-killing) and rubefacient (warming) oil,
rosemary is useful for treating sprains.

- Prepare a compress to which a few drops of
  rosemary oil have been added and apply to the
  injury. Repeat as often as possible to reduce

swelling. Do not massage. Wrap the injured limb in a bandage and rest as much as possible.

- A hot bath (or foot bath if the ankle is sprained) with a few drops of rosemary oil added can help to ease the pain and speed up the healing process.
- Other oils of benefit: lavender, chamomile; arnica ointment is also excellent for sprains, unless the skin is broken.

STRESS

'Stress' is not an illness as such, but a 'multi-dimensional syndrome' which can cause a wide range of physical ailments and psychological problems, ranging from high blood-pressure, headaches or digestive complaints to feelings of constant tiredness, depression or nervous anxiety. Stress also weakens the immune system, and in the long term makes an individual more susceptible to all kinds of disease. Recent research indicates that stress is most probably a causative factor, or a trigger, for many of our so-called 'civilization' diseases such as cancer, ME, stroke, and AIDS. Material proof of the widespread sense of 'dis-ease' experienced today is shown by the high consumption of tranquillizers and stimulants, although it is well known that addiction, a build-up of toxins in the body and other side-effects can be caused by these products if taken regularly. Any treatment which can help to de-stress or revitalize the organism, without producing detrimental side-effects, is therefore of great value.

The possibility of applying new therapies to these wide-spread psycho-neurosis is therefore of considerable importance ... essential oils that are employed in aro-matherapy, in the appropriate doses, are harmless to the organism and do not cause troubles like those produced by the ordinary psychological drugs. Very conclusive experiments in this direction have been carried out in various clinics for nervous diseases, on patients affected by hysteria or psychic depression.[13]

Stress-related problems are an area in which aromatherapy enjoys a great deal of success, due to the powerful combination of touch and smell. During a massage, the essential oils themselves also interact and de-stress the body in two ways: through inhalation (primarily psychological effects) and through dermal absorption (primarily physiological effects). By easing the problem at its source, rather than treating the individual symptoms, aromatherapy is especially valuable for those who suffer from a number of different responses to stress simultaneously. In the words of Dr Ann Coxon:

For instance, a person who has a difficult ongoing life situation, who has high blood-pressure which needs one set of tablets, indigestion requiring another set of tablets, back-pain that would actually be contra-indicated in view of the indigestion, and so on. One could go on with that patient forever. And they invariably end up with 15 pots of tablets, total confusion and a sense of dependency on the doctors. Obviously, the approach of holistic treatment is to help enable people to manage their primary life situation, and the ability of aromatherapy to get at the knot, at the stress reaction itself within the body without using yet more pharmacological treatment is terribly important.[14]

Although stress in often associated with high blood-pressure and restlessness, it can also manifest as a lack of interest in life or feelings of worthlessness or apathy. Rosemary is one of the most useful essential oils for those suffering from the type of stress which results in fatigue, depression and general debility. It acts as a tonic to the whole system and has an uplifting and stimulating effect on the mind. Rosemary is particularly indicated for those suffering from nervous exhaustion after an intense period of mental activity and for those convalescing after a long illness.

• Use rosemary oil in baths, vaporizers, massage and perfumes, for its de-stressing effects.

For specific symptoms, *see* **Debility (Nervous), Depression, Faintness/Dizziness, Low Blood-pressure, Palpitations**.

VARICOSE VEINS
These are the result of poor circulation and inadequate elasticity in the walls of the veins, usually in the legs. The veins become swollen and congested so the blood does not flow back to the heart. Lack of exercise,

standing for long periods, overweight, pregnancy and poor nutrition all contribute to this condition. Rosemary oil can help to improve the circulation, while cypress and rose oils can do much to tone the blood vessels and reduce dilation, although successful treatment does require perseverance.

- General massage or warm (not hot) baths with circulatory stimulants such as rosemary or juniper can help to improve the circulatory system as a whole.
- Make up a massage oil or cream containing rose and cypress oil and rub gently into the area around and above the veins. DO NOT press directly on them or below them, and work up the legs towards the heart. The legs should be elevated after massage. Repeat daily. *See pages 36–7* for instructions on how to make massage oils/creams.
- Other measures: gentle exercise such as swimming or yoga; when possible rest the legs higher than the head; take a course of garlic capsules.

WHOOPING COUGH

Whooping cough, characterized by a sudden intake of breath after a bout of coughing, can develop after a respiratory infection such as a cold, and usually affects children under eight. Rosemary's anti-spasmodic properties have a calming effect and help combat the infection.

- Use in steam inhalations.

- Use rosemary oil in vaporizers in the bedroom, for the course of the illness, and in steaming hot inhalations (to soothe the bouts of coughing).
- Apply a hot compress to the chest using a few drops of rosemary to facilitate breathing.
- Lavender can be used in the same way.

Recipes Using Rosemary

Rosemary Salad Oil

150 ml wine vinegar
3 sprigs of rosemary
1 tsp peppercorns
3 large cloves of garlic
1 red pepper (capsicum)
300 ml virgin olive oil

Boil the vinegar, remove from heat and add the rosemary and peppercorns. Leave to stand for 5 minutes, then remove the rosemary and peppercorns. Grill the garlic cloves and red pepper for about 15 minutes. Remove the garlic skins, and dice the red pepper. Put the garlic, red pepper, peppercorns and rosemary in a bottle and fill with olive oil. Seal securely and leave for 1 week, to allow the flavours to develop.

Rosemary Wine

Queen Elizabeth I was said to have been particularly fond of *Metheglin*, a rosemary-flavoured, alcoholic mead. This is a modern variation:

A handful of 15-cm tips of fresh rosemary

1.8 litres of dry white wine

Soak the rosemary leaves in the wine for 3—4 days, then strain.

Rosemary Tea
Infuse approximately 25 g fresh rosemary in 500 ml very hot water for 5—10 minutes. Strain, then flavour with the juice of half a lemon and honey to taste.

Rosemary Jelly
500 ml rosemary leaves (pressed down)
500 ml water
1 kg cooking apples
500 g sugar
juice of 1 lemon

Simmer the rosemary leaves in the water for 5 minutes. Dice the apples, add them to the rosemary water mixture and boil for 30 minutes. Remove from heat and drain thoroughly (overnight). Add sugar. Boil until jelly sets (about 30 minutes). Skim and stir in the lemon juice. Pour into jars and seal when cool. Serve with cold lamb, chicken or other meat dishes.

If you wish to make this in greater quantities, use 500 g of sugar for every 500 ml of water.

Olives with Rosemary

Black olives
A few cloves of garlic
Strip of lemon peel
Rosemary leaves
Virgin olive oil (to cover)

Put all ingredients in a jar; seal. Leave to marinate for
3–6 months before using.

Rosemary Hearth Cakes

250 g self-raising flour
125 g butter
90 g soft brown sugar
75 g currants
1 egg
1 tbs chopped rosemary

Mix all ingredients into a dough. Roll out and cut into
rounds. Fry over a low heat until golden brown.

New Potatoes with Orange Butter and Rosemary

Toss boiled new potatoes in one part butter, one part
fresh orange juice and a few rosemary leaves (fresh or
dried).

Note:

IF ROSEMARY IS DRIED QUICKLY AT HOME, AND THE

LEAVES STRIPPED FROM THE WOODY STEMS, THEY
RETAIN THEIR DARK GREEN COLOUR.

Marinated Lamb and Rosemary Kebabs
meat from 1 leg of lamb (cut into chunks)

Marinade:
500 g natural (plain) yogurt
4 cloves of garlic (chopped)
juice of 2 lemons
a few rosemary leaves

Marinate the lamb in the marinade mixture for at least
1 hour. Thread the meat onto skewers and grill.

Note:
BOTH ROSEMARY AND GARLIC AID THE
DIGESTIVE PROCESS, AND ARE TRADITIONALLY
COMBINED IN MANY MEAT RECIPES, ESPECIALLY
LAMB AND CHICKEN DISHES.

The Constituents of
Rosemary Oil

Constituent	Percentage
Aliphatic compounds	**0.5–1**
C_5–Aldehydes	(trace)
3–Octanones	(trace)
C–Hexanone	(trace)
3–Octanol	(trace)
Octanol	(trace)
Monoterpenes	**40–55**
α-Pinene	20.25
Camphene	8.10
Myrcene	3.5
β-Pinene	3.7
α-Phellandrene	3.39
α-Terpinene	0.2–0.5
p-Cymene	1.8–2.7
Limonene	3.8–4.7
μ-Terpinene	0.1–0.3
Terpinolene	0.1–0.2
cis/trans-Ocimene	(trace)
δ-3-Carene	0.3–1.4
δ-4-Carene	(trace)
Sabinene	0.4–1.4
α-Thujene	0.07–0.19
α-p-Dimenthylstyrene	(trace)
Bornylene	(trace)

α-Fenchene	(trace)
β-Fenchene	(trace)
Tricyclene	0.34–4.49
Santene	(trace)
β-Phellandrene	(trace)

Sesquiterpenes	**2–6**
Caryophyllene	2–3
Isocaryophyllene	(trace)
α-Humulene	≤1
Cis-α-Bisabolene	≤0.5
α-Copaene	0.15
μ-Muurolene	(trace)
β-Bisabolene	0.04
Ledene	(trace)
μ-Cadinene	0.08
δ-Cadinene	(trace)
α-Selinene	(trace)
α-Cubebene	0.04
Calacorene	(trace)
Cadinene	(trace)
ar-Curcumene	0.17
α-Ylangene	(trace)
α-Muurolene	0.08
trans-β-Fernesene	0.03
Sesquiphellandrene	(trace)
Cadina-1(6)-4-diene	(trace)
β-Maaliene	(trace)
Calamene	(trace)

Terpenoid oxides	
1,8-Cineole	14.4–3.0
Caryophyllene epoxides	(trace)
a-Humulene epoxides	(trace)

Monoterpene alcohols	
Borneol	5.9–9.1
Isoborneol	0.2–0.3

α-Terpineol	0.8–2.1
Cis-β–Terpineol	(trace)
δ-Terpineol	(trace)
Terpinen-4-ol	0.9–1.0
Linalool	0.3–3.5
Geraniol	≤0.1
p-Cymene-8-ol	(trace)
α-Fenchol	(trace)
trans-Sabinenehydrate	0.10
Cis-Sabinenehydrate	0.04
trans-p-Menth-2-en-1-ol	(trace)
cip-p-menth-2-en-1-ol	(trace)
p-Menth-1-en-4-ol	(trace)
p-Menth-1(7)-en-4-ol	(trace)
α-phellandren-8-ol	(trace)
β-Phellandren-8-ol	(trace)
Sabinol	(trace)
cis-Piperitol	(trace)

Monoterpenoid Esters

Bornyl acetate	1–2
Bornyl valerate	(trace)
Isobornyl acetate	≤0.1
Linalyl acetate	≤1
α-Terpinyl acetate	(trace)
α-Fenchyl acetate	(trace)

Monoterpene Ketones

Camphor	15–20
α-Fenchone	(trace)
Verbenone	2–6
Verbanone	(trace)
Carvone	(trace)
α-Thujone	(trace)
β-Thujone	(trace)
Isopinocamphone	(trace)

Benzenoids	**0.5–1**
Phenol	(trace)
O-Cresol	(trace)
m-Cresol	(trace)
p-Cresol	(trace)
p-Vinylphenol	(trace)
Carvacrol	(trace)
Thymol	(trace)
Eugenol	(trace)
Methyl eugenol	(trace)
Trans-anethol	(trace)
Chavicol	(trace)
Methyl-chavicol	(trace)
Safrol	(trace)

R. Tewari and O. P. Virami, 'The Chemistry of Rosemary Oil:
A Review', *Current Research on Medicinal and Aromatic Plants*
[Lucknow, India] 9 (4), 1987, pp. 190–1

References

INTRODUCTION

1. 'Treasury of Botany' quoted in M. Grieve, *A Modern Herbal* (Penguin, 1933), p. 682.

CHAPTER 1

1. *Banckes' Herbal*, cited in *Herbs* (Spring 1995), p. 14.
2. Sir Thomas More, quoted in M. Grieve, *A Modern Herbal* (Penguin, 1931), p. 682.
3. John Brand, 'Popular Antiquities' (1777), cited in *The Herbal Review* (Spring 1989), p. 20.
4. Grieve, *A Modern Herbal*, p. 681.
5. Countess of Hainault to her daughter Queen Philippa of England, wife of King Edward III, in G. Cooper and G. Taylor, *The Romance of Rosemary* (Herb Society/Juniper Press, 1981), p. 16.
6. Cited in R. Le Strange, *History of Herbal Plants* (Angus and Robertson, 1977), p. 215.
7. Brand, 'Popular Antiquities'.
8. Vita Sackville-West, cited in *The Herbal Review* (Spring 1989), p. 21.

CHAPTER 2

1. Cited in M. Grieve, *A Modern Herbal* (Penguin, 1933), p. 682.
2. Cited in G. Cooper and G. Taylor, *The Romance of Rosemary* (Herb Society/Juniper Press, 1981), p. 15.

3. Grieve, *A Modern Herbal*, p. 683.

4. D. Conway, *Magic of Herbs* (Mayflower Books, 1975), p. 137.

5. R. Le Strange, *History of Herbal Plants* (Angus and Robertson, 1977), p. 216.

6. N. Culpeper, *Culpeper's Complete Herbal* (W. Foulsham, 1952), p. 303.

CHAPTER 3

1. Dr J. Valnet, *The Practice of Aromatherapy* (C. W. Daniel, 1980), p. 7.

2. Binet, cited in Valnet, *The Practice of Aromatherapy*, p. 41.

3. R. M. Gattefossé, *Gattefossé's Aromatherapy* (C. W. Daniel, 1993), p. 44.

4. Gattefossé, *Aromatherapy*, p. 38.

5. Valnet, *Practice of Aromatherapy*, p. 41.

6. A. Y. Leung, *Encyclopedia of Common Natural Ingredients* (Wiley, 1980), p. 284.

7. *Database (Aromatherapy)* vol. 2 (Natural Therapies Database UK, 1995), p. 21.

8. Dr M. Lis-Balchin, *Aroma Science: The Chemistry and Bioactivity of Essential Oils* (Amberwood Publications, 1995), p. 92.

9. *Database (Aromatherapy)* vol. 4, p. 21.

10. *Database (Aromatherapy)* vol. 4, p. 19.

11. *Database (Aromatherapy)* vol. 5, p. 15.

12. J. Burne, 'A Spoonful of Oil Makes the Medicine Unwanted', *The Independent*, 30th January 1996, p. 4.

13. Ibid.

14. Lis-Balchin, *Aroma Science*, p. 92.

15. *British Herbal Pharmacopoeia* (British Herbal Medicine Association, 1983), p. 181.

16. J. French, *Book of Rosemary* (HarperCollins, 1993), p. 12.

CHAPTER 4

1. C. J. S. Thompson, *The Mystery and Lure of Perfume* (John Lane, 1927), p. 187; see also J. Lawless, *Lavender Oil* (Thorsons, 1994), p. 4.

2. R. Tewari and O. P. Virmani, 'The Chemistry of Rosemary Oil:

A Review', *Current Research on Medicinal and Aromatic Plants*
[Lucknow, India] 9 (4), 1987, p. 187.

CHAPTER 5

1. Rudolf Steiner, cited in M. Lavabre, *Aromatherapy Workbook*
   (Healing Arts Press, 1990), p. 77.
2. D. Hoffman, *The Holistic Herbal* (Findhorn Press, 1983), p. 81.

CHAPTER 6

1. Dr M. Lis-Balchin, *Aroma Science: The Chemistry and Bioactivity
   of Essential Oils* (Amberwood Publications, 1995) p. 93.
2. *Aromatherapy Quarterly* 40 (1994), p. 36.
3. Alan Barker, 'Aromatherapy and Hepatitis', *Aromatherapy
   Quarterly* 45 (1995), p. 11.

A–Z

1. *International Journal of Aromatherapy* 4 (3), 1992, p. 29.
2. *International Journal of Aromatherapy* 3 (1), 1991, p. 19.
3. *International Journal of Aromatherapy* 2 (2), 1989, p. 7.
4. *British Herbal Pharmacopoeia* (British Herbal Medicine
   Association, 1983), p. 181.
5. P. Davis, *Aromatherapy: An A–Z* (C. W. Daniel, 1988), p. 173.
6. Alan Barker, 'Aromatherapy and Hepatitis', *Aromatherapy
   Quarterly* 45 (1995), p. 11.
7. *International Journal of Aromatherapy* 2 (4), 1990, p. 22.
8. Davis, *A–Z*, p. 293.
9. Davis, *A–Z*, p. 28.
10. D. Hoffman, *The Holistic Herbal* (Findhorn Press, 1983), p. 85.
11. S. Deans and K. Svoboda, 'Aromatics at Auchincruive', *Herbs*
    15 (3), 1990, p. 11.
12. A. Huxley, *Natural Beauty with Herbs* (Darton, Longman &
    Todd, 1977), p. 67.
13. Rovesti, cited in R. Tisserand, *The Art of Aromatherapy* (C. W.
    Daniel, 1989), p. 98.
14. Dr A. Coxon, 'Prescribing Aromatherapy', *Aromatherapy
    Quarterly* 31 (1991), p. 9.

Bibliography & Further Reading

Aqua Oleum, *The Essential Oil Catalogue* (Aqua Oleum, 1994)

T. Balacs, 'Research Reports: Rosemary Inhibits', *International Journal of Aromatherapy* 6 (1), 1994

—, 'Research Reports: Laboratory Shoots', *International Journal of Aromatherapy* 4 (1), 1992

A. Barker, 'Aromatherapy and Hepatitis', *Aromatherapy Quarterly* 45 (1995)

S. Beckett, *Herbs to Soothe Your Nerves* (Thorsons, 1977)

M. Black, 'Dew of the Sea', *Herbs* (The Herb Society, Spring 1995)

British Herbal Pharmacopoeia (British Herbal Medicine Association, 1983)

J. Burne, 'A Spoonful of Oil Makes the Medicine Unwanted', *The Independent* 30th January 1996

Ceres, *Herbs for Healthy Hair* (Thorsons, 1977)

D. Conway, *The Magic of Herbs* (Mayflower Books, 1975)

G. Cooper and G. Taylor, *The Romance of Rosemary* (Herb Society/Juniper Press, 1981)

Dr A. Coxon, 'Prescribing Aromatherapy', *Aromatherapy Quarterly* 31 (1991)

N. Culpeper, *Culpeper's Complete Herbal* (W. Foulsham, 1952)

S. Cunningham, *Magical Herbalism* (Llewellyn Publications, 1982)

Database (Aromatherapy) vols 1–5 (Natural Therapies Database UK, 1995)

E. David, 'The Besprinkling of a Rosemary Branch', *The Herbal Review* (The Herbal Society) 5 (4), 1980

P. Davis, *Aromatherapy: An A–Z* (C. W. Daniel, 1988)

S. Deans and K. Svoboda, 'Aromatics at Auchincruive', *Herbs* 15 (3), 1990

J. de Bairacli Levy, *The Illustrated Herbal Handbook* (Faber & Faber, 1974)

J. French, *Book of Rosemary* (HarperCollins, 1993)

R. M. Gattefossé, *Gattefossé's Aromatherapy* (C. W. Daniel, 1993)

M. Grieve, *A Modern Herbal* (Penguin, 1931)

N. Groom, *The Perfume Handbook* (Chapman & Hall, 1992)

M. Hoadley, *Roman Herbal* (Frank Graham, 1991)

D. Hoffman, *The Holistic Herbal* (Findhorn Press, 1983)

A. Huxley, *Natural Beauty with Herbs* (Darton, Longman & Todd, 1977)

E. Keller, *Aromatherapy Handbook for Beauty, Hair and Skin Care* (Healing Arts Press, 1991)

M. Lavabre, *Aromatherapy Workbook* (Healing Arts Press, 1990)

J. Lawless, *The Illustrated Encyclopaedia of Essential Oils* (Element Books, 1992)

—, *Home Aromatherapy* (Kyle Cathie, 1993)

—, *Aromatherapy and the Mind* (Thorsons, 1994)

—, *Lavender Oil* (Thorsons, 1994)

—, *Tea Tree Oil* (Thorsons, 1994)

—, *Rose Oil* (Thorsons, 1995)

R. Le Strange, *A History of Herbal Plants* (Angus and Robertson, 1977)

A. Y. Leung, *Encyclopedia of Common Natural Ingredients* (Wiley, 1980)

Dr M. Lis-Balchin, *Aroma Science: The Chemistry and Bioactivity of Essential Oils* (Amberwood Publications, 1995)

L. Manniche, *An Ancient Egyptian Herbal* (British Museum Publications, 1989)

M. Maury, *Guide to Aromatherapy* (C. W. Daniel, 1989)

J. Metcalfe, *Herbs and Aromatherapy* (Webb and Bower, 1989)

M. Page, *Herbs* (Frederick Warne, 1980)

A. Percival, *A Nurse's Guide* (Amberwood Publications, 1995)

F. Ransom, *British Herbs* (Pelican Books, 1949)

D. Ryman, *Aromatherapy* (Piatkus, 1991)

C. Stead, *The Power of Holistic Aromatherapy* (Javelin Books, 1986)

R. Tewari and O. P. Virmani, 'The Chemistry of Rosemary Oil: A Review', *Current Research on Medicinal and Aromatic Plants* [Lucknow, India] 9 (4), 1987

C. J. S. Thompson, *The Mystery and Lure of Perfume* (John Lane, 1927)

R. Tisserand, *The Art of Aromatherapy* (C. W. Daniel, 1989)

Dr J. Valnet, *The Practice of Aromatherapy* (C. W. Daniel, 1980)

R. Ypma, *Aroma and Clay Therapy* (The Netherlands: Ogham-Almere, 1993)

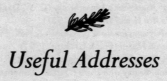

Useful Addresses

It is always advisable to buy rosemary oil from a reputable supplier, to ensure that it is of the highest quality so as to achieve maximum therapeutic results. Aqua Oleum have many years of experience and provide a wide range of top-quality essential oils, including rosemary oil, at very competitive prices. They can be purchased from health and wholefood stores, as well as from some chemists, throughout the UK. Mail-order items, carrier oils, burners, individually formulated products and further information can be obtained from:

Aqua Oleum
Unit 3
Lower Wharf
Wallbridge
Stroud
Glos GL5 3JA
Tel: 01453 753 555
Aqua Oleum also supply
rosemary oil internationally to
the following countries:

Eire

Wholefoods Wholesale
Unit 2D
Kylemore Industrial Estate
Dublin 10

Soap Opera Ltd
Unit 3 Enterprise Centre
Stafford Street
Nenagh
Co. Tipperary

Denmark and Sweden

Urtekram A/S
Klostermarken 20
DK-9550 Mariager
Denmark

Finland

Luonnonruokatukku Aduki Ky
Kirvesmiehenkatu 10
00810 Helsinki

Norway

Terapi Consult AS
Frysjaveien 27
0883 Oslo

USA and Canada

Natura Trading Ltd.
4454 West 10th Avenue
Vancouver V6R 2H9

Hong Kong

The New Age Shop
7 Old Bailey Street
Central

Taiwan

Ecole Internationale
d'Esthetique d'Europe
15F 1 547 Kwang Fiu South
    Road
Hsin Vi Zone
Taipei

Japan

Raiko Co. Ltd.
4B, 2-2-8 Roppongi Minato-Ku
Tokyo

Kawahito Trading Office
Room 308 Fushu Musashino
High Raise 3-11-13
Sakae-cho
Fushu-shi
Tokyo 183

Index